Basic Hospital Financial Management

Donald F. Beck, M.B.A., C.P.A.
Memphis, Tennessee

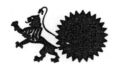

AN ASPEN PUBLICATION®
Aspen Systems Corporation
Rockville, Maryland
London
1980

Library of Congress Cataloging in Publication Data

Beck, Donald F.
Basic hospital financial management.

Includes index.
1. Hospitals—Business management. 2. Hospitals
—Finance. I. Title. [DNLM: 1. Economics,
Hospital. 2. Hospital administration—Economics.
WX197 B393b]
RA971.3.B38   362.1'1'0681   80-19598
ISBN: 0-89443-329-6

Library of Congress Catalog Card Number: 80-19598
ISBN: 0-89443-329-6

Printed in the United States of America

1 2 3 4 5

To Andrea
and to Leslie, Marjorie, and Donald

Table of Contents

Preface

The need for this book became apparent to me when I began teaching college accounting and finance part time. Several colleagues cited a need for a comprehensive book on hospital financial management written by a practitioner. At that time, I was the financial officer of a large medical center and saw a need for a book that could be used to teach persons in the hospital field about financial management. I asked myself these philosophical questions:

If not me, then who?
If not now, then when?

With this book, I attempt to fill that need.

Many individuals were instrumental in assisting me in completing my task. Howard L. Collier read the first draft and made many editorial comments that contributed to the readability of the second draft. Penny Drain typed, retyped, and corrected the manuscript. Completing the project would not have been possible without their help. Finally, I thank my wife, Andrea, for her encouragement and support throughout the book's writing.

Donald F. Beck
November 1980

Introduction

I was pleased when Donald Beck asked me to write an introduction to his book on hospital financial management. Throughout the 60s I was Budget Director and Finance Director for the State of Ohio. The lack of accounting and financial expertise in our nation's hospitals became apparent to many of us at that time. During the 70s hospital financial management became more complex. Government studies, government regulations, the demands of hospital accreditation and of private sector payers often fell upon hospital executives who did not understand this new discipline. Costs grew at an alarming rate.

Throughout this period there was a need for a comprehensive, understandable text. (One wonders if government regulations would be so pervasive and restrictive today if the hospital field had had more financial expertise ten or twenty years ago. Could computer companies have sold expensive hardware and marginally effective software if many hospital administrators had not been desperate?) To help fill this need several adaptations of corporate financial management books were written by academicians.

For the 80s we need books with insight that possibly only a full-time health care practitioner can provide. This book answers that need. The author has written it in the manner he addresses other problems—diligently, intelligently, and pragmatically.

The text contains dozens of tips and numerous examples of insight into the hospital field. It strikes a balance between pragmatism and idealism. One is surprised at the volume of information the book contains because it reads so easily. Anyone with a basic understanding of accounting and an interest in hospitals should benefit from reading this book.

The health care industry is under attack from many sectors and there is cause for concern. We must begin telling our story, and we have a story to tell. There is some risk in explaining health care finance, but better understanding of the field reduces that risk. This book will provide better understanding, and will probably remain relevant throughout the 80s.

Howard L. Collier
Vice President—Finance
Medical College of Ohio
Toledo, Ohio

Chapter 1

Financial Management

The complexity of American hospitals has grown dramatically in the past 15 years. It is commonly recognized that some hospitals in America will be forced to close as this growth in administrative, as well as financial, complexity continues. The chief financial officer will play one of the most important roles in the game of survival. In this chapter we shall see how this position has evolved.

THE EVOLUTION OF FINANCIAL MANAGEMENT

Hospital finance has evolved from a primitive function of bookkeeping/accounting to a role in which it exerts a major influence in the management of hospital assets and the allocation of scarce resources. To help us understand this change, let us look at how the function of hospital financial management has evolved.

Before Government Involvement

Before Medicare, Medicaid, and other widespread government programs, the typical American hospital needed little more than simple bookkeeping. Once a year a decision was made to raise prices. The decision process was not very complex, and a good administrator could easily calculate the needed price increases in less than a day. There was no need for a detailed budget, no need for a cost accounting system, and no cost reports to be filed. Hospitals had the full faith and confidence of the American people. Fund drives were very successful, and philanthropy was common. If money persisted as a problem, the hospital simply raised prices again.

Through the middle sixties, the top financial position was often titled chief accountant or supervisor of accounting. This was sometimes a dependable employee with a high school education and many years of seniority. The supervisor

1

of accounting reported to an assistant administrator, and from 10 to 15 other departments also reported to this position. Accounting was that necessary evil; it did not contribute directly to the hospital's mission in the minds of many administrators, or in the minds of many board members.

The Influence of Government

In 1967 we saw our first Medicare cost reports. These cost reports assumed a cost accounting system that hospitals did not have the expertise to develop. This was followed by Medicaid cost reports. In these early years, the assistant administrator struggled through the cost reports with the chief accountant, or the job was given to independent outside auditors. Neither did a very good job by today's standards; but then the intermediaries were not very astute, so it did not make very much difference.

As the intermediaries became better auditors, the laws and regulations became more complex. The accounting information needs of hospitals grew. Then in 1972 President Richard Nixon signed the Economic Stabilization Act. Clearly, most hospitals were totally unprepared to deal with anything as financially complex as this. Some hospitals ran out of cash. Exceptions were granted to those hospitals that had the most imaginative (and sometimes devious) financial officers. A few hospitals closed. In 1973, the wage and price controls placed on health care by the Economic Stabilization Act were abated. If the price controls had been kept on hospitals for another two or three years, hundreds—maybe thousands—of hospitals would have gone bankrupt.

The Economic Stabilization Act was intended to control inflation. After only a short time, however, wage and price controls were taken off virtually all industries except health care. Health care was singled out as the one industry with an inflationary spiral that needed to be controlled by government for a longer period of time than in other industries in the United States. This was the beginning of a trend that was to throw health care cost into the political arena for years to come. Because the hospital component is the largest component of health care costs—and the component that has the highest likelihood of destroying a person's life savings—it was logical and predictable, even in 1972, that hospitals would experience an increasing amount of government regulation.

In 1977, the Carter administration proposed the Hospital Cost Containment Act, a plan to control hospital revenue that was as complex as the Economic Stabilization Act. President Carter's plan was not approved. For its part, Congress debated not whether hospital costs should be controlled, but in what form these controls should be exercised. Soon after the Hospital Cost Containment Act was rejected, the government announced a program called SHUR. This was an acronym for System of Hospital Uniform Reporting. The federal government published a several-hundred-page SHUR manual as well as extensive reporting forms. The purpose of the SHUR program was to standardize hospital accounting and statistical information. After a more complete analysis, it became apparent that the program would be extremely costly and would not provide the needed comparability between hospitals. At the time of this writing, the SHUR program is no longer considered viable. However, the government is attempting to standardize hospital accounting and statistics through regulations affecting Medicare and Medicaid cost reports. Cost-containment legislation is still being considered by the federal government. In addition, some state governments have passed hospital cost control regulations, and others are considering such regulations. Third party cost reports have never been more complex. Other mandated information requests have never been more numerous. In the 14 years from 1967 through 1980, the financial information needs of hospitals changed beyond recognition. This trend will continue.

THE EVOLUTION OF THE CHIEF FINANCIAL OFFICER

Hospital financial management has evolved into a new dimension. The role of the chief financial officer has evolved into a new dimension as well.

In the sixties, many hospitals that paid for a well-educated, astute chief financial officer were foolishly wasting money. The financial information needs at that time were relatively simple. Today, if the chief financial officer is a green-eyeshade person who ties everything-out-to-the-last-penny, knows every detail in the financial statement, and takes great pride in reporting historical information, then the position is being filled by a person who is grossly inadequate. In other words, if a hospital has the same chief financial officer today that it had in the late sixties, either it was making a mistake then or it is making a mistake now. There are some exceptions to this rule, but, by and large, it is true for the typical American hospital. The evolution of hospital financial management has dictated a role that is more complex. Although many controllers have been able to grow with the demands of the job, many have not.

The future will bring a financial complexity to American hospitals that will cause hundreds to either go bankrupt or sign a contract with a professional hospital management company. Hospital management companies will develop costly financial management programs; but, unlike the independent hospital, they will be able to spread this cost over a large market base. Many hospitals without such resources will just barely survive with barely adequate patient care.

This evolution in the complexity of hospital financial management is totally predictable and logical. It stems from the fact that nothing really important happens in America until industry and labor agree. Thus, on the need for government, as well as others, to control and to regulate health care costs, general agreement between industry and labor has been the major cohesive force.

Most hospital chief executive officers and boards are aware of this evolution. They have been preparing and continue to prepare for the future. In their hospitals, the new position of chief financial officer has been created to fill a void between the chief executive officer and the controller or chief accountant of prior years.

The typical chief financial officer today has many skills that the controller or chief accountant of the sixties did not need. Today's chief financial officer:

- is well educated and has diverse experience;

- has a creative imagination;

- is self-motivated and puts a low priority on blindly following directions from superiors;

- has the interpersonal communication skills to develop participatory cooperation from department heads;

- understands politics, marketing, negotiating, and compromises;

- is more interested in creating future opportunities than in reporting the past;

- and, above all, is a realist.

The details that hospitals needed in the past have not gone away. The chief accountant of the sixties has not been laid off. But the name of the position has been changed to controller or to assistant director of finance. The position no longer reports to an assistant administrator but to a chief financial officer. A whole new level of hospital executives has been created. The chief financial officer now reports directly to the administrator or president. This person is a full-time financial executive to whom few, if any, nonbusiness departments report. The chief financial officer is generally considered the number two person in most American hospitals and has considerably more influence than an assistant administrator.

HOSPITAL GOALS AND OBJECTIVES

The chief financial officer is more concerned with planning creative solutions to problems than with the traditional functions of accounting. The position today demands an individual who understands the changing environment and is willing to master the challenge within the parameters set forth by the chief executive officer and the board. Some hospitals have a formalized statement of goals. Others erroneously believe that the hospital goals are so obvious that there is no need to formalize them. As principal financial advisor to the chief executive officer and to the board, the person who directs the hospital's financial management must fully understand these goals. In this section we will discuss several hospital goals to see how they influence the functions of the chief financial officer.

Social Responsibilities

The social goals of a hospital reflect the institutional commitment to the community it serves. The first component of the social goal defines the level of health care the hospital will provide. Many hospitals should only provide basic services. Some hospitals should provide all general medical and surgical health services. A few institutions are considered major medical centers; their service goals are to provide basic and specialized health services of the highest possible quality. This includes research in the development and application of new patient care methods and an extensive commitment to medical education and research. Each of these levels requires a different financial commitment.

The chief financial officer must direct the hospital's commitment to provide health services to indigents in the local and regional communities. Each hospital should share this burden equitably with other health care institutions. Financial officers can monitor and report indigent care and can recommend policies that define the hospital's commitment. However, the indigent service goals ultimately must be decided by the board.

It is the responsibility of the chief financial officer to ensure that the services offered are those for which an identifiable need exists. Without such monitoring, a hospital might provide costly services that could be provided more effectively in another hospital or outside the hospital setting.

In this era of unfilled wants and scarcity of resources, the input of the chief financial officer in determining the hospital's social responsibilities is extremely important. The benefits gained by achieving a socially desirable goal could be offset either in whole or in part by an accompanying loss in effectiveness in the allocation of total resources.

Financial Stability

Hospitals have an obligation to protect as well as serve patients; to maintain fair prices; to pay fair wages; and to engage in a certain amount of medical education, either formally or informally. Each of these obligations conflicts with the goal of financial stability, at least in the short run. The provision of patient care versus profit maximization, the determination of social justice versus profitable allocation of resources within the institution, and the maximization of care in the most cost effective way are all examples of the fundamental theme of compromise which is found throughout this book. In the following paragraphs, we will examine several specific financial management compromises.

In order to remain financially stable, the hospital must have a policy on rate setting. This includes rate setting for new services as well as annual rate increases. The policy can promote a deficit, a breakeven point, or a specific profit objective by department; or it can promote a specific profit objective that is universally applied to each department. In subsequent chapters, we will learn that all hospitals must have a profit objective to keep pace with inflation and with new technology. The hospital meets this profit objective through application of its rate-setting policy. In an area in which there is more than one hospital, the market serves as a performance index or report card. The physicians indicate how well management is doing in meeting its objective by admitting patients to that hospital that, in the opinion of the physicians, does the best job of maintaining current technology within a reasonable rate structure. In an area with only one hospital, the physicians can still indicate their approval or disapproval of the hospital's support of new technology through rate setting, but in this case it is more difficult to measure.

Another important way in which financial management helps to determine the stability of the hospital is through effective allocation of funds. Nursing wants monitoring equipment, radiology and pathology want new equipment, and the personnel manager wants an expanded fringe benefit package. Decisions concerning allocation of funds in response to each of the requests are in part a result of what the financial manager reports. In developing these reports, the chief financial officer must make the best of an imperfect world. Projections are often upset by external forces over which the hospital has no control. Therefore, sufficient flexibility, such as measures to meet contingencies, must be built into financial forecasts.

If the financial direction of the hospital is too liberal and the hospital experiences a shortage of funds, the results are clear. Vendors not paid in a timely manner are quick to voice dissatisfaction. Employees will not tolerate a delay in payroll. Physical facilities deteriorate because of lack of funds for preventive maintenance and renovation. If the financial management of the hospital is too conservative and the financial manager does not make optimum use of available resources, the results are not as obvious. Nonetheless, the long-term damage to the financial viability of the hospital is no less real by being less evident.

FUNCTIONS OF THE CHIEF FINANCIAL OFFICER

Hospitals differ greatly in size, in ownership, in organizational structure, and in institutional philosophy. The functions of the chief financial officer are influenced by the involvement of the board, whether there is a finance committee of the board, whether there is an audit committee of the board, and by many other factors. This section, therefore, defines the functions of the chief financial officer from a broad perspective. These functions are delineated and treated more fully in later chapters.

Planning

Planning is the most challenging of all financial management functions because it charts where the hospital is going as opposed to where it has been, even though history cannot be ignored. Financial planning is simply a process of expressing an opinion on the future. This opinion is expressed in numbers and presented in a format that facilitates the making of business decisions. It is through planning that the financial person becomes involved in charting the long-run course of the hospital. Without the responsibility for planning, there would be no need for the chief financial officer to participate in professional societies or to attend conferences in health care financial management.

All financial planning begins with an examination of historical data. These data must be prepared in a format or style that closely resembles the format or style being conceptualized for the final decision(s).

The next phase in financial planning is gathering comparative data. Comparative data are often incomplete or otherwise not totally relevant. The gathering of comparable data is often a creative challenge, and success in this task can bring a great deal of personal satisfaction.

Armed with whatever historical and comparative data can be developed, the financial manager is in a position to make an assumption or a series of assumptions concerning the future. The function of planning involves choosing between alternatives and may be formalized in a budget or a report. The final product of planning is nothing more than an informed guess by alert managers who choose between alternatives. In the process of developing significant or long-range financial plans, it is important to build sufficient flexibility into the financing arrangements to cope with unforeseen future developments.

Up to this point we have talked about a process that leads to a decision model. In reality, the process of choosing an optimum decision model and the process of planning for implementation of the particular decision cannot be separated. The fact that most difficult implementation problems are "people" problems and cannot be accurately delineated does not make them less real. An effective financial manager addresses both the analysis and the implementation of any plan as a unified whole. Unless implementation is considered, the plan will present an incomplete picture of the process and the accompanying proposed solution.

Budgeting and financial feasibility analysis are well-known examples of the kinds of planning performed by a financial manager. Another example would be the process of deciding what part of the accounting process could be performed by means of computers and what computer system to use. Could some functions now computerized be done more economically or more effectively by a manual process? Should fixed assets be insured for book value, for replacement value, or for some other figure? Whatever problem the planning process dictates, the four questions that must be answered to arrive at a solution are the same:

1. What has been done in the past?
2. What is the experience of others?
3. Is there a new approach?
4. What is the best alternative to implement?

Organizing

In organizing the financial area of a hospital, the financial manager must keep in mind that nearly all business decisions are interrelated and that the financial team will need the proper conceptual framework to be of optimum value. As a staff function, it is the responsibility of finance to be an advisor and a helpmate.

Goal congruence is the key to a successful hospital organization. Many top management goals, especially in a hospital environment, cannot be justified through sound business reasoning because they are social, humanitarian, or political in nature. If the chief financial officer does not understand the concept of goal congruence, the resulting frustrations will permeate down through the entire business office staff. In a like manner, if one or more of the key supervisors do not understand and accept the importance of organizational goal congruence, it will create frustrations in the minds of many members of the business office staff.

With goal congruence in mind, the manager staffs the financial area with the correct quantity and quality of personnel to carry out the necessary functions. The number of supervisors and the various job descriptions will depend on the size of the hospital as well as the abilities of the individuals involved.

There is an extraordinary number of diverse tasks performed by the business office in today's hospital. It would be futile to rely on job descriptions and on-the-job training to ensure that these tasks are performed timely and uniformly. Each major subdivision of the financial area must have a detailed departmental policy and procedure manual with a description of all known functions. The descriptions of the functions should be detailed enough to enable a new employee to perform the job using the departmental manual as a guide.

In addition to an understanding of goal congruence, department organization, and detailed department policy and procedure manuals, a manager must also be concerned with checklists in organizing the financial area. More than any other executive in health care, a hospital chief financial officer must coordinate many functions through a series of detailed checklists. The interrelated functions in the financial area have a domino effect on each other. When one task is not performed, it affects the efficiency of another task, and so on.

Motivating

In addition to a thorough knowledge of accounting principles and procedures, a hospital financial manager must have a broad general knowledge of the health care industry. This is necessary in order to communicate effectively with and to motivate boards, chief executive officers, physicians, nurses, and other department heads, as well as business office employees. Through informed motivation, department heads will request a reasonable budget and will operate within this budget.

A more specific motivational challenge involves the personnel in the financial manager's own area. The techniques used to inspire enthusiasm in the financial area are no different than the techniques used in any other area of the hospital. The basic principles are to hire people who are intelligent, to always share leadership functions with subordinates, to encourage every employee to be candid with you, and to remember that directors and supervisors have no monopoly on new ideas. These principles are well known, much discussed, and too seldom utilized.

Another very effective motivational technique that is not so well known is to maintain the proper number of employees on the staff. Never allow two people to do what one can do. Overstaffing creates a productivity problem, which in turn creates an apparent need for additional personnel. Before adding to the staff, a financial manager should first study the system to see if greater efficiency and productivity are the answer to a workload problem. This is not to imply that all financial departments are overstaffed or that all workload problems can be solved with a systems improvement. Overstaffing is an easy trap to fall into and a trap that creates morale and cost problems. It is an especially difficult situation that is rarely recognized by the employees.

Controlling

The controlling functions of the chief financial officer can be divided into two major areas: checking and restraining.

Checking functions pertain primarily to the design and the distribution of reports to all levels of management on a routine basis. The most common of these reports are budgets that ideally compare actual performance to a carefully designed standard. In actual practice, the basis of comparison is often a prior-period performance.

The design and continued review of forms is an important function of control. By being alert to the needs of management and by maintaining a thorough knowledge of the health care field, the financial manager can contribute to making sure that the hospital's needs are being met through appropriate forms and records.

The restraining aspect of a chief financial manager's job involves persuasion, investigation, and leadership to channel efforts of department heads and administrators in desired directions. Special reports should be structured to show the most likely outcome of future events. In addition, the financial manager must establish fiscal standards and standards of review for all areas of hospital operations. In order to be most effective, these standards and reviews must be organized in such a manner that they are automatic and ongoing.

SUMMARY

Hospital financial management has evolved from what, by today's standards, was a primitive bookkeeping function into a tremendously demanding and complicated part of hospital management. Much of this evolution has been dictated by government. Government mandates in the future will continue to make health care financial management increasingly complex for years to come.

The role of the senior financial officer and the extent of that executive's participation in financial functions have created the need for a new level in the financial organization of hospitals. The chief accountant of the sixties still exists because the accounting needs of hospitals have not diminished. However, the chief accountant now reports to a chief financial officer who is a central person in the hospital management team. Because of the deep involvement of financial executives in board policy areas, we find this position more and more being viewed as that of a chief executive officer.

The specific role of the senior financial officer will vary from hospital to hospital but can be broadly categorized into four major areas. The first area is planning. Planning is the process of studying history, comparing the present with other institutions, and then expressing an opinion on the future. The second area involves the organization of financial operations to mesh with the goals of the institution and to support these goals as a staff function. The third financial area concerns the monitoring of spending patterns as well as the performance patterns of the hospital. Finally, in the fourth area, the financial manager must perform many control functions. These control functions are broadly categorized into those which check and those which restrain.

DISCUSSION QUESTIONS

1. Describe what influence the government has had on the financial management of hospitals.
2. In what way was the Economic Stabilization Act of 1972 especially significant to the health care industry?
3. What are some of the special qualities to be found in today's successful chief financial manager of a hospital? Contrast this position today with the chief accountant of the sixties.
4. Explain why it is important for the chief financial officer to understand the goals and objectives of the hospital.
5. Explain the differences between the planning functions and the organizing functions of the chief financial officer.
6. Explain several interpersonal skills needed by the chief financial officer of a hospital today. Why are these important?

Chapter 2

General Accounting

Accounting is a function that periodically expresses a set of opinions. These opinions are expressed in numbers that are arranged in neat and exacting formats called financial statements. Most management decisions are based in whole or in part on some accounting report. Therefore, accountants must understand management principles and the needs of management at all levels for numerical data. As hospital management continues to become more complex, accounting must be prepared to play an increasingly important role.

In this chapter we will examine accounting principles and theory in order to understand the basis for the installation and operation of hospital accounting records. We will discuss the preparation and interpretation of accounting reports as well as several statistical reporting functions normally performed by the hospital general accounting section.

CHART OF ACCOUNTS

The fiscal activity of every department in the hospital revolves around and is controlled by the chart of accounts. The hospital's chart of accounts is considered in the design of forms, in all procurement functions, in systems design, in report preparation, and throughout the budgeting function. The chart of accounts is the most universally used document in the hospital.

Definition

The chart of accounts is an elaborate, precise set of abbreviations. In order to insure flexibility, to make interpretation simple, and to produce financial reports in an expedient manner, these abbreviations are expressed in numbers rather than in letters.

To understand why we need this set of abbreviations, let us examine how transactions would be handled without a chart of accounts. Assume the radiology department payroll includes three classifications of salary expense. These are: technicians, clerical, and other. On the last day of the pay period, this department has three kinds of revenue: inpatient revenue, outpatient revenue, and professional fees. The department also purchases supplies, film, and a piece of capital equipment. Without a chart of accounts, the financial transactions in this simple example would be recorded as follows:

Debit
Radiology salaries—technicians
Radiology salaries—clerical
Radiology salaries—other
Social Security expense
Other fringe benefits
Radiology inpatient accounts receivable
Radiology outpatient accounts receivable
Radiology professional fee accounts receivable
Radiology supply expense
Radiology film expense
Movable equipment
Credit
Accrued salaries payable
Federal withholding payable
Social Security payable—employee
Social Security payable—employer
Other fringe benefits payable
Radiology inpatient revenue
Radiology outpatient revenue
Radiology professional fee revenue
Accounts payable
Cash

The above example shows the excessive amount of time it would take to enter the description of all the accounts in this simple case. The magnitude of entering actual account descriptions for the thousands of transactions that occur in a hospital would be staggering. In addition, it would require an enormous computer to accept and accumulate transactions by their full description. It should be clear that an elaborate, precise, logical, and structured set of abbreviations is necessary. The hospital chart of accounts, expressed in numerals rather than in alphabetic letters, becomes the needed set of abbreviations.

Illustration

The chart of accounts for any organization must be tailored to suit that particular entity. To illustrate, we will develop a chart of accounts for a medium-sized community hospital. We must caution that this illustration is not a suggested chart of accounts. In reality, a hospital is much more complicated than the example, and the reporting demands placed upon hospitals by outside agencies require a more involved chart of accounts.

In our example, assume the hospital has a general fund, a plant fund, an endowment fund, a loan fund, and a self-insurance fund. (The principles of fund accounting are explained in the following section.) Whenever a transaction is initiated, we must determine which fund is affected. There are presently five major funds. The first question we ask is whether there will ever be more than ten different funds. It appears unlikely, so only one digit will be set up to indicate the correct fund. The identifying digits will be:

- 0—general fund
- 1—plant fund
- 2—endowment fund
- 3—loan fund
- 4—self-insurance fund.

It has now been established that any account whose first digit is zero (0) will be a general fund account, any account whose first digit is one (1) will be a plant fund account, and so forth.

Within each fund the two major statements will be a balance sheet and a statement of receipts and expenses. Assume that it has been decided that it is unlikely there will ever be more than one thousand different balance sheet, receipt, and expense types in the aggregate. Therefore, three digits are assigned to this classification of account.

The balance sheet represents the continuing permanent accounts of the hospital. Account numbers for these accounts would, therefore, be assigned first. The major balance sheet categories are: current assets, long-term assets, current liabilities, long-term liabilities, and fund balance or equity accounts. Numbers are assigned as follows:

- 100–149—accounts in the current asset section
- 150–199—accounts in the long-term asset section, including accumulated depreciation
- 200–249—accounts in the current liabilities section
- 250–274—accounts in the long-term liability section
- 275–299—accounts in the fund balance or equity section.

Up to this point, we have identified an abbreviation to designate which fund is being affected, and we have identified ranges of numerical abbreviations to designate balance sheet accounts within these funds. The next task is to assign ranges of numerical abbreviations to the statements of receipts and expenditures. For the general fund, the statement of receipts and expenditures is the income statement. Since the general fund is the most comprehensive and the most used fund, numbers are assigned to fit the income statements. Categories in the other fund statements of receipts and expenditures will then be designed to conform with this assignment of numbers. Assume numbers are assigned as follows:

- 300–349—room and board revenue
- 350–474—ancillary revenue
- 475–499—outpatient revenue
- 500–574—allowances and contractual adjustments
- 575–599—other revenue.

As expense account numbers are assigned to revenue departments, care should be taken to ensure that these expense accounts follow the same pattern assigned to revenue accounts. For example, if revenue for nursing station four north is 312, then expenses for nursing station four north should be 612. If revenue for radiology is 440, then expenses for radiology should be 640. This relationship will make the chart of accounts easier to use. With this in mind, expense account numbers are assigned to all the revenue producing departments as follows:

- 600–649—nursing department expenses
- 650–774—ancillary department expenses
- 775–799—outpatient department expenses.

Other department expense numbers could be assigned as follows:

- 800–824—administrative service expenses
- 825–899—general service expenses
- 900–974—plant services expenses
- 975–999—miscellaneous expenses.

By using four numerical digits, the particular hospital fund as well as the hospital department can be identified. Numbers must still be assigned to identify detailed type of revenue by department and detailed type of expense by department. The numerical abbreviation to identify detail within a department is referred to as the standard object code. Assume that this field will require three digits and that groups of numbers have been assigned as follows:

- 0–99—detail identifying type of revenue
- 100–199—detail identifying type of revenue deductions
- 200–299—salaries and wages
- 300–349—fringe benefits
- 350–399—payroll taxes
- 400–599—supplies
- 600–799—services
- 800–899—other operating expenses
- 900–949—depreciation expense
- 950–999—miscellaneous.

Our chart of accounts parameters are now complete and can be summarized as follows:

Digit	Description
1	Applicable hospital fund
2–4	Balance sheet, income, or expenditure type
5–7	Detail of revenue or expense item

The next step is to assign specific numbers to the different items within these parameters. Although the example used to develop this chart of accounts was hypothetical, the process is identical to that used by all hospitals in establishing and maintaining their charts of accounts.

Use

Accounting must support constantly changing organizational objectives. The chart of accounts represents the hub around which many of the accounting functions revolve. The chart of accounts, therefore, must be flexible enough to shift with changes in organizational structure, managerial objectives, available resources, and internal as well as external reporting requirements. In addition, the person maintaining the chart of accounts must be familiar with the uses of general ledger information and with accounting principles.

Assignment of new chart-of-account numbers and deletion of account numbers no longer required should be centralized and performed by one person, such as the supervisor of accounting. In the absence of the supervisor of accounting, the controller should be responsible for approving changes in the chart of accounts. Under no circumstances should the director of purchasing or any other department head be authorized to make such changes. A department head is not familiar enough with the multiple uses of the instrument. It should also be cautioned that, in a medium-sized or large hospital, the chief financial officer is too far removed from the detail to approve changes in the hospital's chart of accounts.

All departments use the chart of accounts to obtain account numbers for purchase requisitions, to analyze monthly budget as well as other department operating reports, and to accomplish other tasks. Therefore, each department should be issued a new updated chart of accounts at least annually. Large departments should be issued more than one copy. Also, at least annually the accounting department should conduct workshops in the use of the chart of accounts. These workshops should be attended by department secretaries, new employees, clerks, and others who are responsible for assigning account numbers on the various hospital forms and requests. These workshops can be scheduled just before the hospital begins its annual budget process.

Updates to the chart of accounts should be distributed on a timely basis following a carefully defined policy and procedure. In this way, department personnel are informed when a new account affecting their department has been established.

FUND ACCOUNTING

We will not deal here with the principles of general accounting. It is assumed that the reader already has some knowledge of basic accounting principles. However, most hospitals have more than one fund. Fund accounting is usually ignored in basic accounting texts. In this section, therefore, we will explain some principles of fund accounting and will define the most common funds used by American hospitals.

Principles

An accounting fund is a sum of money or other assets that have been segregated in order to carry on a specific purpose, attain a particular objective, or fulfill a specific purpose. Funds can be established by charter, by board action, by law, by bond indenture, by restrictions on a grant or a gift, or by other action.

A separate hospital fund requires a separate self-balancing set of accounting records. For example, assume a hospital is given one million dollars with the stipulation that the principal or corpus of one million dollars remains intact. Interest earned on investment of this money can be used for any of three purposes: equipment for the newborn nursery, hospital care for premature infants born to indigent families, or for neonatal research projects. It would be very difficult to comply with all of the restrictions placed on this gift if the money were comingled with the hospital's regular income and expense accounts. The money is therefore placed in a separate restricted funds bank account and accounted for through a restricted funds set of accounting records. Since the number of transactions in the restricted fund account are few, it will not be difficult to ensure compliance with the restrictions of the gift.

Funds are established for several specific functions in the hospital. It is important from an accounting point of view to regard each fund as a separate enterprise. Since each fund is viewed as a separate business established for a specific purpose, it will have its own complete set of accounting records. A controller should never make a journal entry in which the debit is to the general ledger of the hospital and the credit is to the general ledger of one of the hospital's suppliers. Similarly, a controller should never make a journal entry in which the debit is to the hospital general fund and the credit is to another fund of the hospital. Each entry in each fund should be a complete self-balancing transaction in which debits equal credits. This is an important point to remember. Most errors with hospital fund accounting occur because accountants fail to view the different funds as separate entities and proceed to make entries in which the debit is to one fund and the credit is to another fund.

To illustrate proper fund accounting, assume a check is written on the general fund account to pay for a restricted fund expense. The transaction should be:

General Fund
Debit: Due from restricted fund	$X.XX
Credit: Cash	X.XX

Restricted Fund
Debit: Expense	$X.XX
Credit: Due to general fund	X.XX

When the transfer of cash is made to reimburse the general fund for this transaction, the proper accounting is as follows:

General Fund
Debit: Cash	$X.XX
Credit: Due from restricted fund	X.XX

Restricted Fund
Debit: Due to general fund	$X.XX
Credit: Cash	X.XX

General Fund

All hospitals, as well as other business entities large enough to require a general ledger, have a general fund. Although it is not always necessary to have additional funds, most hospitals do in fact have one or more funds in addition to the general fund.

The general fund is used to record the hospital's day-to-day activities. Most of the income and expense entries will be recorded in the general fund. The only transactions not recorded in the general fund are those that are required by law or by administrative policy to be accounted for separately.

Plant Fund

The plant fund, now becoming common, is used to record all property, buildings, equipment, and depreciation. Depreciation is normally recorded as a general fund expense, and cash is transferred to the plant fund at regular intervals.

The majority of the plant fund detail consists of departmental listings of equipment that show tag number, description, date acquired, original cost, accumulated depreciation, estimated useful life, and any other information required by the hospital to comply with external reporting requirements. The plant fund also has the majority of the hospital long-term debt, mortgages, and any reserves required by the debt instrument. Construction-in-progress work orders should also be recorded in the plant fund.

Endowment Fund

Often a hospital will inherit or be given cash or other properties under conditions that stipulate that income produced by such resources may be used to benefit the hospital. The original principal is not expendable and must remain intact. When the uses of fund income are restricted to certain activities, the endowment is called a restricted endowment. When no restrictions are placed on the use of fund income, the endowment is referred to as an unrestricted endowment. Income from unrestricted endowments is available to the general fund.

Some hospitals have only one or two endowments to account for. In this case, the endowments are normally in the restricted fund rather than in a separate endowment fund.

Endowment funds pose a very unique and often complicated custodial function for accounting purposes. If the hospital has several endowment funds, it becomes difficult to properly account for them in a normal restricted fund; in this case, a separate self-balancing endowment fund should be established. Some hospitals transfer all endowment money and other assets to the trust department of a bank. The bank will professionally manage the investment of the fund principal and transfer income earned back to the hospital.

Loan Fund

If the hospital has a teaching program, it may have loan funds. Loan funds consist of money that is available for loans to students. The students may be in nursing, in laboratory or radiology technology, or in other paramedical areas. Loan funds may come from government grants, from gifts, from interest income accumulated over a period of time, or they may be established by board action.

If the hospital has only one or two small loan funds, they can be accounted for through a restricted fund account. As the amount of loan fund activity increases, it becomes more expedient to establish a separate loan fund.

Restricted Fund

The restricted fund is used to account for any resources on which restrictions have been placed either by the donor or by the hospital governing body. The loan fund and the endowment fund are used for specific purposes. The resources in a restricted fund are more general; such funds are often restricted for such diverse needs as the acquisition of medical resources or a medical library; the purchase of a specific piece of equipment; or the establishment of a specific new service, nurses training, distinguished lecturer honorariums, or other activities.

In accepting restricted funds, the hospital must be very careful. If the funds are accepted to initiate a major new service, a study should be performed to determine how this new service will fit into the overall, long-range role and program of the institution. The hospital also should carefully study the effect of accepting restricted gifts on third party reimbursement. Most restricted fund receipts must be offset against the hospital's operating expenses with only the net amount being reported as an allowable expense for Medicare and Medicaid cost reporting. The hospital is not required to offset unrestricted receipts. Through careful planning, the hospital can maximize cost reimbursement. Often, in accepting unrestricted funds, the hospital can promise to make every attempt to satisfy the wishes of the donor. Unrestricted funds offer more planning flexibility and do not reduce third party cost reimbursement.

Self-Insurance Fund

Many hospitals are self-insured for part of the coverage needed. Although most self-insurance funds are established to settle malpractice claims, there is nothing to preclude self-insurance for fire, employee bonding, workmen's compensation, liability, or for any other insurance need. The self-insurance fund may be established for a single hospital, or it may represent the efforts of several hospitals that have pooled their resources in order to self-insure the group for a specific need.

The annual amount of money to be transferred to the self-insurance fund to cover liability claims for a specific purpose should be determined by an actuary or other professional. Self-insurance must be entered into cautiously. In addition to the risk exposure incurred by the hospital, there are several complicated third party payer reimbursement problems to be resolved.

Other Funds

The funds described here do not represent a complete list of all the funds that might be established. Hospitals have established funds for such diverse purposes as annuities, retirement of indebtedness, construction in progress, and for other specific permanent or temporary purposes. The number of funds used by a hospital corresponds to the specific needs of that particular enterprise. Whenever a particular accounting need or legal requirement becomes difficult to maintain, the hospital controller can consider establishing a new fund. It is important to remember that each fund is treated as if it were a separate and distinct accounting entity. Neither hand-posted nor computer-generated journal entries should be made which affect more than one fund. Debits, by fund, should always equal credits by the same fund.

ACCOUNTING REPORTS

The accounting department of an enterprise is responsible for compiling and distributing many reports. Hospitals are no exception. Because the nature of the accounting reports must fit the unique characteristics of the particular institution, in this section we will examine accounting reports from a general perspective.

Design of Management Reports

Accounts have a general tendency to produce too much detail for reporting purposes. This is especially true in hospitals that have electronic data-processing capabilities. Some feel that if you give an individual a large stack of printouts that contain all possible detail, the accounting responsibility has been discharged. The fallacy of this approach lies in the fact that each individual has a comprehension level that is determined by interest, time, authority, and other factors. If people are given detailed reports that exceed their comprehension level, then they have been given nothing. Indeed, some reports are so full of detail that even fiscally oriented department heads will not spend the time needed to utilize them.

In designing a report, the accountant must first understand the viewpoint of the nurses, technicians, tradesmen, and department heads. There is an inverse relationship between the amount of authority and the need for detail. A person with a wide span of authority requires a minimum amount of detail. A person with a narrow span of authority requires a wide base of detail to manage effectively. This relationship is depicted in Figure 2–1.

First-line supervisors need more detail than assistant administrators in order to manage effectively their areas of responsibility. An assistant administrator, in turn, needs less detail than a department head but more detail than an administrator. A board member should never be given more than a one- or two-page summary rounded to the nearest thousand dollars.

In designing a management report, one often hears the complaint that "the administrator will not explain what is needed" or "if the department heads would just tell me what they want, I could get it for them." However, users of such reports cannot be expected to understand what their needs are until they understand what information is available. It is the responsibility of the controller to direct the design of reports. The process is similar to checking the spelling of a word in the dictionary. You may not know exactly how to spell the word, but when you see it you instantly recognize it. The administrator, department heads, and others do not know exactly how to design a report to provide the needed information, but when they see it they instantly recognize it as something they want and need.

When the controller designs management reports, it is not enough to tell the facts and to give supporting information. The controller must also accept responsibility for the user's understanding and conclusions. More discussion on types of reports as well as illustrative examples are included in the chapters on budgeting.

Figure 2–1 Authority Versus Need for Detail

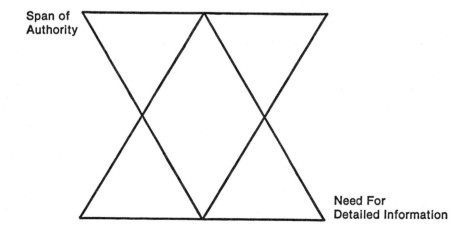

Timing of Reports

Accounting reports may be prepared daily, monthly, quarterly, or annually. A daily report should be prepared showing at least cash receipts, cash disbursements, cash balance, gross revenue, and patient days. Other information monitored on a daily basis will depend on the needs of the particular hospital. Monthly reports include a balance sheet and an income statement for the general fund and at least a balance sheet for each of the other funds. Departmental budget reports are also prepared monthly. These are discussed in more detail in the chapters on budgeting. In addition to the monthly requirements, the hospital will prepare several additional reports at year end. All of these reports must be prepared on a timely basis according to a regular and consistent schedule. If the reports are not timely, they have decreased value. If the reports are not distributed on a regular and consistent schedule, they will not be used. In the following paragraphs, we present some thoughts on how to reduce the time required to issue reports.

Department heads realize that corrective action must begin as soon as possible. Because of the increasingly complex requirements placed on department heads, better and faster closing techniques are being demanded. The most effective tool to minimize closing procedures is a closing schedule. This schedule must be prepared monthly and distributed to every employee who plays a part in closing, even if that part is small. The closing schedule should include the following information: the function to be performed, the name of the employee who will be responsible, the day of the week, and the time of day to the nearest half hour. The schedule should be determined in consultation with the employees and should be changed from month to month if necessary. Through careful scheduling, the hospital gains the advantage of having every move toward closing timed as early as possible in relation to other moves. In addition, by publishing the employee name rather than title, the plan is personalized in that all employees know the when and the why of their particular role. The schedule becomes a standard with delays subject to exception reporting. Some hospitals might consider distributing the results each month after closing has been completed.

Two other important steps can be performed before month end to expedite closing. The first is to summarize and prepare recurring journal entries, especially those for fixed charges or for accruals that will be reversed. The other is to prepare in advance working papers and report forms in which available comparative figures can be inserted. It is poor accounting to cut off transactions earlier than the end of the period. However, by preparing workpapers and reports as completely as possible ahead of time, one can significantly reduce the time required to close.

Accounts payable, revenue, and other large-volume transaction areas should employ interim summaries and accumulations. For example, accounts payable can be summarized on the last or second-to-last day of the month, with a supplementary journal entry set up to record late invoices.

Many administrators receive preclosing reports of key summary information. Techniques of forecasting are worked into these reports, and these techniques can be refined over a period of time. These estimates will be surprisingly close to the actual results that will be finally reported several days later. The estimates have the advantage of giving administration an extremely quick look at the results of operations. They also provide the basis for a validity check on actual statements before their final publication.

Other General Accounting Functions

The accounting department will receive many requests for checks to be prepared for use in payment for goods or services received or for use in transferring cash from one fund to another. An approved policy and procedure must be followed in approving these requests and in preparing the checks. A check request form is the starting point in the process. The request form should contain at least the following information: the date, the name and address of the person or firm the check should be made payable to, the purpose for which the check is drawn, the account number(s) against which the check will be charged, a box to indicate whether the check should be mailed directly or be returned to the department making the request for subsequent forwarding, and a place for authorized signatures. A hospital policy and procedure manual should contain the full description of the hospital policy on checks that do not flow through the normal accounts payable system. If the hospital does not have a policy and procedure system, the policy should be explained completely on the back of the request form.

Another function of the accounting department is the signing of all checks. Most hospitals have a signature plate and some form of mechanical check signing. The signature plate must be kept in a locked, secure place. A log should be kept that lists in numerical sequence all check numbers that have been endorsed. Voided checks must also be accounted for. This log should be kept for each fund and compared against cancelled checks on a regular basis.

All hospitals are required to keep logs on Medicare, Medicaid, and other third party payer revenue. These logs are very detailed, require a large amount of time, and must be kept current. If the logs are not prepared by a data-processing system, a 36- to 40-column pad of paper is required. All third party revenue logs should be summarized at least semiannually. Quarterly summaries are preferable. In addition to revenue logs, third party payer cost reports require a mass of other statistical data, such as pounds of laundry processed for hospital departments and housekeeping assigned hours. Often the same person who is responsible for the revenue logs will also be responsible for maintaining the supplemental statistical data required for the Medicare, Medicaid, and other third party payer reports.

The hospital accounting records will probably be subjected to from two to five outside audits per year. Before each audit the key personnel in the accounting department should discuss the objectives of the audit, who will coordinate the audit, and how closely the work of the auditors will be monitored. If it is the annual audit by the hospital's independent outside auditors, the work of the auditors does not need to be monitored very carefully. If it is the annual audit by the hospital's Medicare intermediary, the activities of the auditors must be monitored very closely, especially with respect to information solicited from department heads.

The activities examined in this section represent only part of the many diverse activities performed by the accounting department. Other general accounting functions include responsibility for the correct account numbers on requests and forms, special studies, requests for information, monthly outside reports such as hospital administrative studies, completion of government forms, and tabulation of various statistical data on departmental activities.

SUMMARY

The hospital chart of accounts is an elaborate, precise set of numerical abbreviations. It is the center of all accounting activity and must be carefully designed as well as updated to meet the changing requirements of the particular hospital. In making changes to the chart of accounts, the reporting and information needs of the hospital must be considered. In this chapter we have presented the design of a chart of accounts to illustrate the careful reasoning that underlies this function.

Hospitals use fund accounting principles in order to separate different objectives or to fulfill specific purposes. Funds can be established by charter, by board action, by law, by bond indenture, by restrictions on a grant or a gift, or by other action. Each fund should be considered a separate and distinct business entity for accounting purposes. Each accounting entry in each fund should be a complete self-balancing transaction in which debits equal credits.

All hospitals have a general fund in which day-to-day income and expense transactions are recorded. In addition, the hospital may have one or more other funds, such as a plant fund, endowment fund, loan fund, restricted fund, self-insurance fund, or other fund. The number of funds used by any hospital is determined by the accounting needs or policy requirements of the particular hospital.

Accounting reports should always be user oriented. There is a general tendency among accountants to provide more detail than necessary. If a report exceeds the comprehension level of the person receiving the report, then it is as if the person were given nothing. First-line supervisors need and can comprehend more detail than the administrator.

To have maximum benefit, accounting reports must be timely. The most important tool used to speed up closing is the closing schedule. Other techniques are summary journal entries, advance preparation of working papers and report forms, interim summaries and accumulations, and preparation of preclosing reports.

DISCUSSION QUESTIONS

1. Explain the purpose of the hospital's chart of accounts. How does the chart of accounts fulfill this purpose?
2. List several uses of the chart of accounts.
3. Explain the use of a fund in fund accounting.
4. What are some ways in which a hospital fund can be established? How is the number of funds determined?
5. Define general fund, plant fund, and restricted fund.
6. What points should be kept in mind when designing management reports? Explain.
7. How can the amount of time required to close an accounting period and to prepare the required financial reports be shortened?
8. List several functions of the hospital accounting department.

Chapter 3

Payroll Accounting

All hospital employees are experts when it comes to monitoring their own paychecks. Employees demand exactness as well as timeliness and are quick to register a complaint if an error is found. It is generally agreed that a good payroll department exemplifies accuracy and scheduling.

OBJECTIVES OF THE PAYROLL SYSTEM

The modern hospital payroll department has three main objectives. These are to meet critical due dates, produce accurate information, and satisfy records retention requirements.

Meet Critical Due Dates

The cost of being one-half day late with an employee payroll is extremely high. The cost of being an entire day late with a payroll is disastrous. Due dates for filing various payroll withholding and payroll tax reports are also critical since the penalties for late filing are usually very high.

Every payroll department should maintain a critical due-date list. This list is prepared before the beginning of the fiscal year and is updated or revised at the beginning of every month. An example of a critical due date list for Community Hospital is shown in Table 3–1.

The critical due-date list can be prepared to show weekly dates. The list should show enough detail to clearly identify all required due dates. As a function is completed, a line is drawn through it. At the beginning of every week, the chief financial officer should review the status of the critical data file with the supervisor of payroll.

Table 3-1 Community Hospital Critical Due Dates

Month Ended April 30, 19X1

Function	Target Date	Due Date
Final input of data for biweekly payroll	April 2	April 2
Pay distribution to employees	April 7	April 7
Deposit part of payroll in bank	April 7	April 7
Deposit part of payroll in bank	April 8	April 8
Collect time cards from departments	April 14	April 15
Final input of data for biweekly payroll	April 16	April 16
Pay distribution to employees	April 21	April 21
Deposit part of payroll in bank	April 22	April 22
Complete form 941, employee withholding and F.I.C.A.	April 23	April 30
Complete state income tax withholding	April 23	April 30
Complete city income tax withholding	April 23	April 30
Complete state unemployment tax	April 25	April 30
Complete and deposit special federal estimate	April 29	April 30

Produce Accurate Information

Various federal, state, and local laws require the accumulation of certain specified data by employee, by pay period, by month, by quarter, and so on. To comply with these laws, the payroll department must create a detailed and accurate data base. This data base must be capable of producing information to satisfy diverse information needs.

In addition to complying with government regulations, the payroll department is responsible for accurately distributing over 60 percent of the hospital's expenses. Accordingly, safeguards must be provided to ensure that payments are in accord with management's general plans and specific authorizations. Accurate payroll data are used by the hospital to maximize reimbursement from third party payers. These records are also useful in labor negotiations, budget preparation, and rate reviews.

Satisfy Records Retention Requirements

Payroll records must be retained for specified periods of time and be available for inspection by those responsible for enforcing laws and regulations. These time periods are much shorter than most hospitals realize. For example, the Fair Labor Standards Act and the Code of Federal Regulations specify the following retention periods:

Type of Record	Required Retention
Payroll checks	Two years
Earnings register	Three years
Payroll register	Three years
Labor cost records	Three years
Employee withholding	Four years

Many payroll managers feel that they must keep all original records for at least a certain time. Six years is quoted most often. In fact, most payroll records can and should be destroyed before six years. It has been estimated that 65 percent of the money spent for records retention is wasted and that hospitals never refer to 85 percent of their records.

On the other hand, it must be remembered that pay is used to determine rights to accumulated vacations, sick leave, and retirement benefits. The hospital's annual payroll register showing year-to-date information should be kept for 50 years. Most hospitals microfilm this information in order to reduce the retrieval time as well as filing space.

In summary, it can be stated that record-keeping policies must be guided by the rule of reason and the probability and dollar amount of risk involved, not by statutes of limitations alone.

EMPLOYER PAYROLL TAXES

Many years ago, only the employer and the employee were involved in payroll transactions. The bookkeeping problems were relatively simple because an employee who earned $100 received $100 on payday. Today, the problems of accounting for payroll are staggering. The required accounts and supporting documents required by federal, state, and local governments have caused the clerical expenses of accounting for payroll to rise rapidly.

Employer/Employee Relationships

Persons performing services for the hospital may be generally classified as either employees or as independent contractors. Payroll systems are concerned only with employees and the records associated with employees.

For payroll tax purposes, an employee is generally considered to be anyone performing services subject to the will and control of the hospital. This general rule applies even though the hospital permits professional employees considerable discretion and freedom of action. The hospital—through its board of directors, medical director, or administration—has a legal right to control the result of employee services and can discharge an employee.

Individuals in business for themselves are not employees. Professional fees paid to outside auditors, consultants, physicians, tradesmen, and others who perform services contracted for by the hospital are not considered as payments to employees. Payments to outside contractors are not subject to employer payroll taxes. It should be noted that the hospital saves considerable fringe-benefit expense in addition to employer payroll taxes if the person performing the service is not classified as an employee.

For payroll tax purposes, there is generally no distinction between classes of employees. Superintendents, managers, other supervisory personnel, and hourly personnel are all employees. If an employee/employer relationship exists, wages paid to the employee are subject to all payroll taxes.

Social Security

Unless the hospital is part of a state government or a political subdivision, Social Security taxes are normally paid on all employees. The rate and maximum amount of wages subject to Social Security per employee change often. Most hospital payroll systems account for the maximum amount subject to Social Security as well as the correct rate.

Certain payments to employees are not considered wages subject to Social Security. The exempt payments can be substantial, and the hospital will overpay Social Security taxes if a system to identify exempt payments is not carefully monitored.

Some examples of payments to employees that are not subject to Social Security taxes are:

- certain specified payments to nonimmigrant alien students, scholars, trainees, teachers, and others

- deceased worker's wages paid to a beneficiary and disabled worker's wages if made in a calendar year after the worker was deceased or was disabled

- reimbursement for employee moving expenses

- retirement, pension, and workmen's compensation payments

- many sick payments made by a hospital

- payments to student nurses.

Federal Unemployment Tax

The federal unemployment tax is imposed on employers and cannot be deducted from employees' pay. At the time of this writing, the effective federal unemployment tax rate is 0.7 percent of the first $6,000. This rate is arrived at by taking the 3.4 percent federal rate less a state unemployment tax credit of 2.7 percent. State ratings below 2.7 percent reduce dollar for dollar the total amount of unemployment tax paid, since the federal government allows a credit equal to 2.7 percent even if the state rating is below that amount.

Workmen's Compensation

Workmen's compensation insurance or tax is calculated on gross earnings paid. Workmen's compensation is generally paid quarterly or semiannually. Usually, the hospital can accept the rate calculated by the state or can become a part of a group insurance plan. The group plans generally have a lower rate and can save substantial expense. The state hospital association would have information on possible workmen's compensation group insurance plans.

Workmen's compensation rates are subject to merit reductions. Therefore, many hospitals treat minor injuries in their own emergency rooms, employee health centers, or other facilities. By not reporting these incidents, a hospital can effect a favorable experience rate. The employee is professionally treated, and the hospital contains costs.

State Unemployment Tax

State unemployment tax on employers may vary from 0.2 percent to 4.0 percent depending upon the applicable state rating system. At the time of this writing, most state unemployment rates applied to only the first $6,000 of gross wages paid per employee. State unemployment tax returns are filed quarterly.

TYPES OF REMUNERATION

All hospitals have at least two types of remuneration that can be generally classified as salaried and hourly. Many hospitals also have an executive payroll that offers special perquisites and benefits.

The salaried payroll includes those employees who receive a specified amount of pay per month as opposed to an hourly rate. The salaried payroll includes most supervisory personnel and often includes secretaries, administrative assistants, and other administrative personnel. The pay received by salaried personnel is not dependent upon hours worked.

Hourly personnel receive a specified pay rate per hour. In addition, the hospital normally has an evening shift differential and a night shift differential. The hourly payroll is further complicated by requirements to pay an hourly premium for overtime, for work performed on holidays, and in some job classifications for work performed on weekends. Total hourly pay, then, is a function of time worked (often computed in tenths of an hour), hour of the day worked, day worked (i.e., weekend or holiday), and established hourly pay rate for the particular person performing a particular function. Although the logic is simple, the sheer magnitude of calculations required to compute the hourly payroll makes it impossible to compute manually. Virtually all hospitals have some system of electronic data processing for the hourly payroll. The payroll department must prepare and verify the data input, monitor the computer output, and process the numerous changes required in the data memory bank.

The chief executive officer and other key supervisory personnel are often classified in an executive payroll. This payroll normally has special perquisites and fringe benefits. To guarantee the confidentiality of the executive payroll, it is normally processed by the hospital's independent outside auditors or by the chief financial officer, rather than through the payroll department.

Some hospitals grant bonus- or profit-sharing plans in addition to base salary. These incentive plans provide additional compensation for performance that is superior to or equal to some predetermined objective. Incentive plans vary widely in their detail, in their application, and in the number and types of employees eligible.

FRINGE BENEFITS

In the past ten years, the value of fringe benefits has been increasing twice as fast as the average pay for time worked. This growth of fringe benefits has improved employee wellbeing but has not had a noticeable effect on improving employee motivation. Fringe benefits are perceived as a condition of employment and an integral part of the total compensation package.

Paid Vacation Days

Most hospitals have two paid-vacation policies, one for hourly personnel and another for salaried personnel. The policy for hourly personnel normally corresponds to the number of years of continuous service. The hourly vacation policy should have a carefully prepared addendum to define vacation accrued for part-time employees. For personnel on the salaried payroll, there is often no correlation between length of service and number of vacation days.

The payroll department must insist on well-defined vacation and other days-off policies prepared by personnel or by administration. Employees attempt to accumulate as many vacation days as possible by taking holidays, compensatory time off, sick days, or other days off whenever possible. It is the responsibility of the payroll and personnel departments to minimize abuse of days-off policies. To accomplish this task, the personnel in payroll must be acutely aware of established policy and must constantly watch for attempts to substitute other paid days off for vacation days.

The hospital policy that either prohibits or limits vacation carryover from year to year is defined by the personnel department but carried out by the payroll department. An established policy is necessary to regularly identify those employees who may lose accrued vacation days if they do not take time off. These incidences must be reported to the employee as well as to the department head.

Holidays and Other Paid Days off

The number of paid holidays has been growing with most hospitals granting eight or more defined days off and one or more floating holidays. The floating holiday may accrue on the employee's birthday, the beginning of the hospital's fiscal year, the employee's anniversary date of hire, or some other time. It is important that the hospital have a carefully defined policy on accrual of floating holidays.

Other paid days off are governed by the hospital's prevailing practice for jury duty, witness duty, military leave, and bereavement. Virtually all hospitals have a policy granting paid time off for jury duty, witness duty, and bereavement. Many also grant some paid leave (other than vacation) while fulfilling annual military reserve obligations, which are usually two weeks in duration. This leave is not extended to employees who are drafted or enlist for a regular term of military service.

Although most hospitals have a policy defining other paid days off, it is the responsibility of the payroll manager to ensure that these policies are detailed enough to be administered without bias.

Insurance

The three most common types of insurance coverage offered by hospitals are hospitalization and medical insurance, life insurance, and salary continuation or long-term disability insurance.

The provision of some type of hospitalization and medical insurance for full-time employees is universal in American hospitals. About half of the hospitals also offer this benefit to part-time employees. A growing majority of hospitals pay 100 percent of the premiums, some pay half of the premiums, and others pay between one-half and all of the premiums. Dependent coverage is also universally offered, with most hospitals paying all or part of the dependent premiums.

While nearly all hospitals provide life insurance as a fringe benefit, the amount and kind of coverage varies widely. At the time of this writing, only the cost of group term life insurance up to $50,000 is considered a fringe benefit. The cost of group term life insurance in excess of $50,000 provided to the employee is considered ordinary income, and the payroll department must provide the employee with a statement showing the amount of ordinary income to report at year end. Similarly, any group or individual permanent life insurance premiums paid by the hospital are ordinary income unless the right to permanent insurance or equivalent benefits is forfeitable if the employee leaves the job. Any ordinary income must be calculated and reported by the employer. It is the responsibility of the payroll department to comply with internal revenue service regulations concerning the reporting of miscellaneous ordinary income derived through the hospital's payment of insurance benefits.

Long-term disability coverage must be carefully defined in order for the payroll department to determine eligibility and to prorate premium expense. The hospital long-term disability coverage can be contributory or noncontributory. The policy may cover only full-time employees, only supervisory personnel, or all hospital personnel including part-time employees.

Pension and Annuity Plans

Approximately two-thirds of the hospitals provide a noncontributory pension plan. The hospital's annual contribution is actuarially determined, and the payroll department is not involved. For the one-third of the hospitals that provide a contributory pension plan, the payroll department must calculate and deduct the employee contribution.

Most nonprofit hospitals offer an optional tax-sheltered annuity program. If the hospital contributes any matching amount to the employee contribution, this matching amount is calculated through payroll records. If the hospital does not provide any matching contributions, the payroll department must deduct only the applicable amount from the employee's gross wages and from the employee's statement of earnings (federal Form W-2) at year end. The amount deducted is forwarded to the underwriting insurance company. Some hospitals limit tax-deferred annuity plan options to a single insurance underwriter to control clerical cost, while other hospitals permit employees to engage in annuity plans with a large number of insurance underwriters.

The regulations concerning current taxability of amounts withheld for tax-deferred annuity are often different for state and local income taxes. The payroll department is often required to calculate wages net of annuity for federal withholding reporting and to calculate wages before adjusting for annuity contributions for state and local withholding reporting.

Sick Leave

The majority of hospitals allow 12 paid days of sick leave per employee per year. Some organizations allow unused sick-leave days to accumulate indefinitely, some provide incentives for not taking sick-leave days, and some allow sick-leave days to accumulate to a specified maximum. In addition to performing the clerical functions of accounting for sick-leave days taken or accumulated by an employee, the payroll department must attempt to recognize and report attempted abuses of the sick-leave policy.

It must be cautioned that with sick leave as well as other personnel matters, the payroll department should enforce but should not determine hospital policy.

Other Fringe Benefits

Other fringe benefits include employee discounts, tuition assistance, meal-discount programs, special cash awards, annual physicals, and uniform allowances. The involvement of the payroll department in administering these benefits depends upon the particular hospital policy defining the benefit.

EMPLOYEE DEDUCTIONS

In addition to levying employer taxes, the local, state, and federal governments require that the hospital act as a collection agent. In addition to government-mandated deductions from employee earnings, the hospital will have many other employee deductions.

The employees in the payroll department must be familiar with the laws of taxation and withholding because the hospital is subject to significant penalties for failure to comply with government withholding regulations.

Social Security

Most nongovernment hospitals are required to withhold a portion of the earnings of each employee for Social Security. Some state and federal government hospitals do not withhold Social Security but are required to deduct for a specific government pension plan.

Amounts withheld for Social Security are the employee's contribution to the combined federal programs for old age and disability benefits, Medicare, and survivors benefits. Employers are required to withhold at a specific rate on earnings up to a specific amount. The schedule of tax rates and the maximum amount subject to tax are revised frequently by Congress. These changes generally have no effect on the general components of the payroll system.

Income Tax Withholding

The largest employee deductions are for employee income tax withholding. The amount required to be subject to federal withholding varies in accordance with the employee's marital status, number of exemptions, and estimated deductions and credits the employee will claim when filing the annual income tax return.

In addition to federal income tax withholding, many state and local governments require employees to withhold income tax from employee wages. The determination of the amount to be withheld varies among the different states and local government units. Many hospitals employ personnel from more than one state. In this instance, the payroll system must be flexible enough to accommodate the withholding requirements of multiple state regulations.

Other Deductions

In addition to compulsory deductions from gross earnings for payroll taxes, there are many other deductions authorized by employees or the unions representing the employees. The list of other potential deductions includes, but is not limited to, pharmacy or other employee purchases, life insurance, health and major medical insurance, union dues, savings bonds, united fund contributions, other charitable contributions, tax-deferred annuities, and contributory pension plan amounts. It is important that the payroll department have the proper signed authorization for each deduction. If the authorization for deductions is kept in the personnel department, then the payroll manager must insist on a signed internal communication from the personnel department authorizing each deduction.

PAYROLL ACCOUNTING SYSTEM

The necessity for accuracy and the amount of detail generated by the payroll functions require complex systems and subsystems. In this section, a relatively uncomplicated system is outlined in order to show the major components. In actual practice, a hospital payroll system requires many supporting subsystems.

Input Data

As shown in Figure 3–1, the payroll system requires three basic types of input data for each pay period: constant data, the accumulated earnings record, and variable input. Constant data include such information for each employee as name, address, social security number, income-tax withholding data, rate-of-pay and other data from the hospital's position control roster, and general ledger account numbers to be charged. Constant data also include social security tables; federal, state, and local withholding tables; unemployment-tax maximum earnings amounts; authorized deductions; pension-plan calculations, if applicable; and other data that remain relatively constant from pay period to pay period.

Figure 3-1 Payroll System Flow Diagram

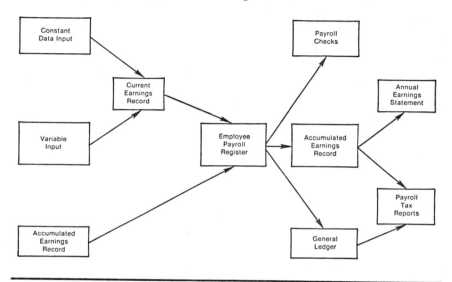

Variable input includes data that are unique to the individual pay periods. These are: hours worked, time of day worked if shift differential applies to the position; vacations, sick leave, or holidays taken; and applicable employee deductions (i.e., pharmacy purchases, pay advances, garnishments).

The constant data input and the variable input are matched together to compute the current earnings record. In studying the payroll department workflow, audit checks, and systems design, it is important to recognize that there are two separate types of input data and that each has its distinct characteristics.

The updated earnings record includes all payroll information that is being accumulated on an annual basis. Some data will be accumulated on a calendar year basis, some will be accumulated on the hospital's fiscal-year basis, and some must be accumulated on both a fiscal year and a calendar-year basis. In designing or improving the payroll system of a hospital whose fiscal year does not coincide with the calendar year, it is important to determine the output requirements and then to design a system to satisfy these requirements. It is often mistakenly assumed that information cannot be accumulated on both a fiscal year and a calendar-year basis.

Employee Payroll Register

The current earnings report and the accumulated earnings report together make up the current pay period employee payroll register. The employee payroll register is the focal point of a good payroll system. All payroll systems should pivot around the employee payroll register. Its design varies in accordance with the number and kinds of fringe benefits, classes of employees, number and kinds of deductions, extent to which automation is used, and type of equipment available.

The employee payroll register should be the only mechanism through which the hospital's accumulated earnings record and actual payroll expense accounts in the general ledger can be updated. Accruals and other balance sheet journal entries can be made, but direct payroll expense accounts should be changed only through the payroll register. Otherwise many hours will be spent tracing information through a system with an inadequate audit trail.

Output Information

The employee payroll register is used as the data base to generate payroll checks and employee payroll earnings reports that generally show year-to-date as well as current-period gross earnings, detailed deductions from earnings, and net earnings. The payroll register is also used to generate an updated accumulated earnings record and to post to the hospital general ledger. The accumulated earnings record must be generated on a calendar-year basis but may also be generated on a fiscal-year basis.

The accumulated earnings record is used to produce the required individual annual earnings statements for employees as well as for federal, state, and local governments. The accumulated earnings record and the information from the general ledger are used to produce required payroll tax reports.

PAYROLL SYSTEM CONTROLS

Payroll systems are very complex because of the considerable volume of data required and the mass of computations needed. If precautions are not taken, one person alone can easily manipulate a payroll. Even with proper safeguards, the possibility of collusion between two or more employees makes fraud comparatively easy.

Separation of Duties

To prevent collusion, to avoid padding of the payroll, and to facilitate the work of the various persons in the payroll department, the duties of the employees involved in hiring of personnel, the computation of payroll, and the disbursement of payroll should be separated as much as it is practical to do so.

It is often not practical to separate completely the computation and disbursement of payroll. However, some separation is necessary and can be accomplished easily, even in a small hospital. For example, all hospitals can separate the disbursement of checks and the monthly reconciliation of the payroll checking account. This is accomplished by making the accounts payable personnel responsible for the reconciliation of the payroll bank account. The payroll department in turn should be responsible for the reconciliation of the hospital's general bank account.

Dual data files should be maintained for all employment authorizations, rate changes, job classification changes, and terminations of employment. One data file will be maintained in the payroll department, and a second file will be maintained in the personnel department or in administration if the hospital is too small to have a separate personnel department. At least once a year, and ideally more often, a complete employee payroll register should be compared with the detail contained in the dual data file. This audit must be unannounced. The mechanics of the audit are relatively simple and can be performed by a temporary-help person if the hospital does not have the nucleus of an internal audit function.

Payroll Disbursements

Because of the volume of payroll checks, most hospitals use mechanical equipment to sign checks. The signature plates or rubber stamp pads should be under the control of one person. A numerical accounting of all checks signed as well as all checks voided should be maintained by this person. This person should immediately investigate any break in the numerical sequence of check numbers maintained in a log.

Unclaimed payroll checks should not be kept under the control of the payroll department. After a reasonable period of time, all unclaimed payroll checks should be turned over to another department, such as personnel, cashiers, general accounting, or administration. The identity of persons who call for these checks should be carefully verified. Payroll checks that remain unclaimed over a long period of time should be turned over to the hospital's independent outside auditors, internal auditors, or chief financial officer. These checks will require a careful investigation and followup.

Employee terminations generate another special problem. When an employee terminates, it is easy for a fellow employee to continue to clock the terminated employee in and out. It is also easy for a supervisor to accept and cash the continuing paychecks received for a terminated employee. To prevent these and other attempts to defraud the hospital, a well-planned procedure for terminating employees must be approved. This procedure should include an investigation of subsequent payrolls to verify the removal of terminated employees. This investigation should be made by someone independent of the payroll department.

Timing of Payroll Cash Needs

All hospitals must strive to maintain noninterest-earning cash balances at the lowest possible level. Excess cash should be maintained in temporary investments or other current assets. In the chapter on cash management, it is shown that cash can easily be invested for as short a period as two days.

Compared to other industries, hospitals have a relatively high ratio of employees whose income represents the second income for their households. These include not only part-time and temporary employees but many full-time employees as well. Because of this, the timing between disbursement of payroll and receipt of the check for payment at the hospital's bank is generally significantly longer than in other industries.

By studying the monthly payroll account bank statements, the hospital can determine the pattern of time delays between disbursement of checks and debits against the hospital's bank balance. This time pattern should be computed for both early-in-the-week pay periods and for pay periods that fall near a weekend. Once this pattern can be predicted with reasonable accuracy, the hospital can play the "bank float." The cash can either be placed in temporary investments or used for other purposes until the funds are needed to honor employee paychecks.

The hospital must carefully foster bank relationships or negotiate in advance a procedure to handle a situation of insufficient funds in the payroll bank account. The hospital must also guard against seasonal fluctuations, such as a tendency to cash paychecks more quickly during the Christmas shopping season.

In addition to using the bank float on employee net-pay distributions, the hospital has several other opportunities to maximize its use of cash through the payroll system. Employee withholding, as well as employer and employee Social Security amounts, are generally not required to be deposited until the third banking day after the end of the quarterly period. One-quarter monthly periods end on the 7th, 15th, 22nd, and last day of each month. Many state and local taxes or withholding amounts are not required to be deposited until the end of the following month or the end of a calendar quarter. With careful planning, a hospital can significantly affect its use of cash by delaying payroll taxes and payroll withholding amounts as long as possible without incurring a penalty.

SUMMARY

The three major objectives of a payroll department are to meet critical due dates, to produce detailed and accurate information, and to satisfy records retention requirements. A very complex set of systems and subsystems are required to satisfy these objectives.

Federal government requirements include employer and employee Social Security, unemployment compensation, and employee income tax withholding. State requirements include workmen's compensation, unemployment compensation, and, in many states, income tax withholding. In addition to these government-mandated requirements, the hospital payroll department must satisfy hospital-controlled payroll-related needs. These include insurance, vacations and other days off, pension and annuity plans, other fringe benefits, and employee deductions.

The payroll system input data include constant data, variable data, and accumulated earnings records. The employee payroll register is the focal point of the system. Because of the vast amount of detail required, payroll systems are vulnerable to employee fraud and abuse.

The payroll system offers the hospital an opportunity for temporary investment because of the timing between pay distribution and debit against the hospital bank account.

DISCUSSION QUESTIONS

1. Explain why the need for accuracy in payroll is so critical.
2. What is the difference between an employee and an independent contractor working for the hospital?
3. Name the major federal and state employer payroll taxes.
4. Discuss three common hospital fringe benefits.
5. What are some of the characteristics of the different types of input data required by a payroll system each pay period?
6. Define the employee payroll register.
7. Explain one of the major problems associated with payroll disbursements.
8. How can hospitals promptly distribute payroll checks and at the same time temporarily use the funds for investments?

Chapter 4

Billing and Cashiering

In this chapter we will follow a patient bill from admission through receipt of payment. Patient billing and cashiering includes many highly variable tasks and periods of time. In addition, hospitals vary widely in type of automated equipment used, flow of paperwork, and manner of billing. In the following sections, we will examine the broad tasks and functions that are applicable to all patient revenue systems.

INITIATING THE PATIENT BILL

The patient revenue process begins in the preadmission or admission effort when a primary financial class is assigned to the patient. This financial class is sometimes called an insurance code; it includes such classifications as Medicare, Medicaid, county welfare, Blue Cross, other commercial insurance, indigent compensation, workmen's compensation, selfpay, and other forms of payment. In addition to a primary financial class, most patients will be assigned a secondary financial class that indicates the responsibility for charges not covered by the primary payer. As soon as the patient is registered, the admitting office transmits the information to the billing section for verification.

The financial class or charging status initially entered into the system is subject to change. Often patients are unaware of the fact that they have only partial coverage or that their policy has a deductible portion. Often when the hospital attempts to verify coverage there is a denial of benefits. New information may be collected that alters or changes the financial class. Proper identification of the financial class is a key element in the patient billing system. It is important that the verified charging status be properly reflected in the system and that changes be entered as soon as practical if the hospital is to remain financially solvent.

In addition to collecting proper billing information, it is important that the admission procedure code contains enough data to perform good quality business research. For example, every hospital should do a patient-origin study periodically. Studies are often required on patients admitted by age or diagnosis. Seasonal admitting patterns or studies of admissions by physicians are often requested. If the hospital has electronic data processing, the basic problem is that of getting accurate input information into a format that can be entered into the computer without the cost of expensive manual conversion steps after the point of origin. If the hospital utilizes a manual system, the basic problem is to make sure that at the point of origin all information needed to prepare billing as well as analysis reports is collected.

Two basic practices are often utilized to enhance the quality of information collected in the admission process. The first is to train admitting personnel to ask questions in such a manner that they are understood by the patient. For example, the patients should be asked if they are responsible for a portion of the bill, not asked if they have a coinsurance and deductible clause in their policy. If the patients do not know which government program they are on, the admitting clerk should ask what day of the month the check normally comes in the mail. If the check arrives on the third of each month, it is probably Social Security; if the check arrives on the first of each month, it is probably a welfare program; if the check arrives later than the third day of the month, it is probably a pension check. By phrasing questions from the patient's point of view rather than in the vernacular of hospital billing personnel, the admitting clerk can obtain more accurate information, and at the same time the patient will feel more comfortable and less threatened.

Another technique commonly used to enhance the collection of admitting information is a periodic in-depth review of the admission form and the admission procedure to simplify the process and save total personnel time. Hospital billing requirements are undergoing a constant change as third party payers become more demanding and more aggressive. A formal review of all forms used in the admitting and billing process should be made annually and whenever a change is made in the hospital's equipment used in the patient revenue process.

LOST-PATIENT CHARGES

Every hospital experiences some problems with lost-patient charges. Because most cost contracts limit reimbursement to the lower of cost or charges, it is important to minimize lost-patient charges for Medicare, Medicaid, and other cost-reimbursed programs as well as for those patients who pay billed charges.

Departmental Responsibility

Patient charges for radiology, laboratory, and other ancillaries flow from nursing stations or clinics, to the department responsible for the service, to either data processing or the business office. Throughout this flow of paperwork, the ancillary revenue center should be made responsible for ensuring that all legal charges get into the billing system. This is important because, if the responsibility is not clear, it is often assumed that the user center is responsible and the system ultimately breaks down. In some institutions, it is the responsibility of the business office or data processing to get all patient charges into the billing system. The business office can process all charges that are sent from departments, but it can do very little to identify charges that never enter the system.

The department rendering ancillary services should keep a log book to record all patient services. Department directors should receive adequate reports that enable them to monitor gross revenue generated by their department on a daily basis. For example, if pharmacy floor stock or items from a central supply exchange cart are given to a patient but no charge ticket is initiated, the system must enable the director of pharmacy or the director of central supply to identify the nursing station where the lost charge initiated. The item is then charged against the budget of the nursing station responsible. Often a patient charge cannot be initiated because the supply was wasted. Wasted supplies are supplies that are unusable and nonchargeable but need to be replaced. User departments should process a waste tag that is put through the system that charges the item to the budget of the user department.

If a patient charge ticket is incomplete or illegible, it should be returned to the area where it originated. Often the area that originated the charge is a nursing station or other user department. In this case, the ancillary department must be made aware of the returned charge tickets so they can follow up on this potentially lost revenue with the relevant department. If the ticket cannot be corrected, the cost of the lost item or service should be charged to the cost center where the charge originated.

Administrative Responsibility

It is the responsibility of hospital administration to make sure that nurses, aides, clerks, orderlies, technicians, and others understand the significance of lost charges. In some hospitals, the prevailing attitude and concern is based solely on patient care, with no realization that patient care is not possible without a system for billing. The concept that charging is very important must be stressed in orientation and periodic inservice training programs. Although one patient may benefit from an unrecorded charge, other patients are penalized by a corresponding increase in the amount they are required to pay for the service they receive. Unless the personnel in the departments that perform the patient care realize how lost tickets affect the hospital, there is little chance of success in implementing improvements in the system.

The hospital also has a responsibility to make sure the billing system is practical. Whether the system is manual or fully automated, it is considered practical if human participation is not complex at the nursing stations and in the ancillary departments. The most important technique used to simplify the charging system is to have a uniform charge requisition form for every major service. A wide range of size and style in forms for recording charges must be avoided. Other techniques that can be considered to simplify the charge system include but are not limited to: "mark-sense" charge plates to put data simultaneously in both human and machine language, coded labels on each charge item that can be transferred to a patient card, pharmacy drug exchange boxes for use in anesthesia, and automatic pricing done by computer.

Regular and periodic lost charge audits should be conducted by someone in the billing or accounting area. This person should have sufficient knowledge of the charge collection procedure to address adequately the potential for revenue enhancement. If the hospital maintains a serially numbered control of charge slips in the revenue producing departments, the audit should include a test of these numbers. A test can also be performed to correlate departmental statistical data with recorded revenue. The most common, and normally the most accurate, lost-charge audit technique is to review a sample of final bills against the patient medical records. Because of legal and accreditation requirements, medical records' charts are normally accurate.

Patient Bed Census

In addition to charges for ancillary services, the hospital must carefully monitor the patient census. The most common errors are:

- Patients admitted through the emergency room close to midnight are assigned a bed but often are not charged for the day if they are in surgery when the midnight census is taken.

- Maternity patients admitted and assigned a bed are often in the labor room when the census is taken and thus not charged for the day.

- Transfers are sometimes recorded as discharges.

- Patients that expire are often not discharged on the census system.

Errors in billing for patient days are significant because of the amount of the charge. Normally, the per-day room rate is equal to several ancillary charges.

Cost of Lost Charges

It is important to minimize lost charges. However, it should be understood that all hospitals experience some lost charges. Furthermore, it would be foolish to invest in a system to reduce lost charges if the system costs more than the potential cash benefit. To calculate the probable cost of lost charges on the potential for cash gain by reducing losses, the hospital must know the percentage of cost-reimbursed gross charges and the percentage of bad debts and free care. Since these classes of patients are not affected by the hospital charges or prices, little cash benefit will be gained by reducing the number of lost charges for services performed on such patients. The following formula can be used to estimate the percentage of net revenue that will be gained for the hospital from every dollar of reduction in lost charges:

$$PI = 100 - (CR + BD + FC)$$

where   PI = Percent increase in net revenue
           CR = Percent of revenue that is cost reimbursed
           BD = Percent of revenue that is bad debt
           FC = Percent of revenue that is free care

To illustrate, assume a hospital is 60 percent cost reimbursed, bad debts are 5 percent of revenue, and free care is 3 percent of revenue. The percent of revenue gained by reducing lost charges is:

$$PI = 100 - (60 + 5 + 3) = 32 \text{ percent}$$

In this case, if the hospital were to reduce lost charges by $100,000, it could expect to gain $32,000 in cash. At the same time, contractual adjustments would increase $60,000, bad debts would increase $5,000, and free care would increase $3,000.

It should be noted that the above calculation assumes the hospital charges are equal to or greater than the hospital's cost as defined by the most liberal cost-based third party payer. If the hospital's cost reports indicate that customary charges are substantially less than costs, the percent of revenue gained by reducing lost charges is:

$$PI = 100 - (BD + FC)$$

In this example, if the hospital were to reduce lost charges by $100,000, it could expect to gain $92,000 in cash. This is because cost-based third party payers normally pay the lower of cost or charges; and, until charges are equal to or greater than cost, the hospital can increase reimbursement by increasing charges either through price increases or by reducing the number of lost charges.

INTERIM BILLING AND DISCHARGE PROCEDURE

When the patient is admitted, a file or folder is initiated that contains all the information obtained in either the admitting or preadmission process. This information is verified as soon as practical so coinsurance, deductibles, and non-covered charges are known before the patient is discharged.

Interim Billing

If the patient has been in the hospital for a week, an interim review should be made to make sure that all billing information is complete and verified, claim forms and assignments have been signed, and arrangements have been made for personal items such as telephone, private room differential, and television. An estimate should be made at this time of the amount of liability the patient will have at discharge. This amount should be studied in conjunction with credit and employment information obtained from admitting. A judgment can then be made whether to send interim bills while the patient is still in the hospital. Some hospitals prefer to call the interim bill a report of progress. If interim bills are to be sent, it must be decided whether the patient or someone in the patient's family will receive the bill. Sometimes the physician can help in making these decisions.

Discharge Procedures

It should be an established nursing policy to notify the business office as soon as the patient's date and time of discharge is known. Usually the date of discharge is known at least the day before. It is especially important to have many of the names of those patients who are to be discharged early near the end of the week or the day before a major holiday, when the number of discharges is unusually large.

The discharge clerk calculates the estimated patient liability for all scheduled discharges. This includes personal items such as private room differential, television, and telephone. The patient is also responsible for coinsurance, deductibles, and noncovered charges. Occasionally the patient's insurance will pay 100 percent of the hospital bill, or arrangements will have been made in advance to pay small noncovered charges. If this is the case, the nursing station can be notified that the patient is not required to stop at the business office. All other patients must have a discharge pass that is issued by the business office when a family member makes arrangements for payment. If the patient is not a courtesy discharge and does not have a discharge pass, the nursing station must make sure the patient stops at the discharge desk before leaving the hospital.

The hospital's chief financial officer should establish a maximum dollar amount that the discharge clerk can handle. If the estimated patient liability exceeds this established limit and the patient is not in a position to pay the amount due at the time of discharge, the discharge clerk should direct the party to the credit department. Some hospitals have established for the discharge clerk a dollar limit for those patients who express a willful nonsettlement, a second limit for those who indicate an inability to pay, and a third limit for those who will not settle the balance at discharge because they believe there are significant errors or omissions in the estimated bill.

It should be understood by the discharge clerk that this is a routine policy and in no way reflects on the credit standing of the patient. It is necessary to take a firm position with some patients, but this posture should always be taken in the credit office and not at the discharge desk. The credit office must have a private room in which the patient can be interviewed.

The hospital should clearly inform the patient that the bill received at discharge is tentative and should be settled at that time. The patient should also be informed that another bill will be mailed within two weeks. When patients indicate they will send a check to the hospital, a return envelope should be provided. It has been proven that return envelopes speed collection.

THE BILLING FUNCTION

We have followed the patient revenue system from admission through the hospital stay and finally through the patient discharge. In this section we will examine the hospital billing function.

Billing System Maintenance

The billing department will have an insurance screen or billing master for prorating charges and for bill preparation. If the hospital uses electronic data processing, this can be programmed into the computer. If the hospital has a manual billing system, the insurance masters are outlined in the department procedures manual or directives. The hospital should have an established insurance master for Medicare, Medicaid, two or more of the most common Blue Cross coverage options, and any other major third party payer. The insurance masters should be monitored on a regular basis and undergo a formal review at least annually.

Cost-based third party payers do not pay billed charges. Instead they pay either an interim rate based on a percent of billed charges or a per diem amount or level periodic payments based on a forecast. Whichever method is used by cost-based payers to make interim payments, a careful review is needed at least quarterly. It is to the hospital's advantage to negotiate an interim rate that overpays and requires the hospital to refund money through the cost report. It is to the third party payer's advantage to negotiate an interim rate that underpays the hospital and results in a lump sum settlement when the cost reports are finalized. It is important to be aware of this fact when interim rates are reviewed and negotiated.

The third part of the billing system that requires regular review is the number of days between discharge and the sending of the bill to the patient or third party payer. After discharge, the patient account is normally kept open to allow for late charges. Late charges are patient charges or credits that reach the business office after the patient has been discharged. If the charge system is working smoothly, three or four days is ample for posting late charges. If the charge system has paperflow problems, the hospital may have seven or eight hold days. The number of days a patient account is kept open before a final bill is produced should be formally reviewed at least annually.

Processing Patient Bills

The billing system produces a detailed bill that subtotals charges by revenue center. The billing department must first review the itemized bill for reasonableness. The purpose of this commonsense review is to determine whether the charges appear reasonable for the diagnosis. For example, a woman in maternity should have a delivery room charge. If a baby was delivered, there should be a nursery charge. If surgery was performed, there should be a recovery room charge and substantial central supply charges. Most serious malfunctions in the billing system will be discovered in these commonsense reviews.

After this review, the bills are ready to be sent. The patient should always get a complete copy of the itemized bill. Some third party payers require a copy of the itemized bill while others only require a summary. Many third party payers insist on an itemized bill as well as summary charges transferred to their tailormade statements. For Medicare, Medicaid, and other cost-based third party payers, a summary copy of each patient bill must be sent to a clerk responsible for posting the revenue logs. Complete procedures for each type of billing should be in the departmental policy and procedures manual, which is available to all billing persons.

If the patient has insurance coverage, some hospitals wait until the insurance portion has been paid before billing the patient for his portion. It is not uncommon for some insurance companies to wait two months before paying a claim. In this case, the patient would get no notification for two to three months. It is far better to estimate the patient portion of the charges and bill immediately or to send the patient a statement for the entire amount at the same time a statement is sent to the insurance company. If the hospital is overpaid, a refund check can be prepared. In addition to being more advantageous to the hospital's cash flow, experience has shown that collections are significantly greater if the patient receives a statement at the time the initial bill is sent to the insurance company than if the patient is sent a statement for the balance after the insurance company or other third party payer has paid.

As noted earlier, late charges are billable services that are delayed. These charges reach the business office after the original bill has been sent. If the charges are significant, a supplemental bill should be prepared and sent to third party payers as well as to the patient. If late charges are relatively small, they should be written off to an adjustment account rather than billed.

Hospitals sometimes have special arrangements with physicians, other hospitals, clinics, and others to process diagnostic tests. For example, physicians might send all of their lab tests to the hospital for processing under an agreement that a statement be prepared once a month. Special arrangements represent unique problems, and it is important that responsibility for billing these charges be clearly delegated and understood.

The initial billing should be followed up with a second bill within three to four weeks. This procedure should apply to third party payers as well as selfpay accounts. Sometimes a commercial account has to be followed up as frequently and as diligently as a chronically slow individual payer.

Timing of Patient Bills

It is false economy to reduce the number of personnel in the billing section to a level at which it is not possible to achieve timely billing. Even in a small hospital the cost of being one week behind in inpatient billing is equal to or exceeds the salary of an employee. Therefore, it is important to have enough staff or enough backup to ensure total daily submission of every billable account and to work constantly at minimizing unbillable accounts. One technique used to provide backup for the billing department is to have floaters who rotate from credit and collections to billing. The personnel responsible for posting the third-party payer revenue logs can rotate to the billing function during peak periods, but this must be done cautiously since the revenue logs must remain current.

Many hospitals staff the billing department during the night hours. Others employ many part-time personnel in billing. Part-time personnel can more easily work extra hours during peak periods, accept temporary layoffs more readily than full-time personnel, and require far fewer fringe benefits than full-time personnel. Whichever techniques are employed, it is important to make sure that the billing supervisor has an adequate pool of staff to call upon as needed.

Different classes of patients have different seasonal hospital utilization trends. In order to provide the staffing flexibility to bill on a timely basis throughout the year, new personnel in billing should be trained in all phases of billing. With rotation of duties, adequate training, and careful orientation to the entire hospital, a new person should be able to bill all classes of payers—including Blue Cross, Medicare, Medicaid, and other third party payers—within six months.

One person on either the medical records budget or the business office budget should be responsible for utilization and insurance coordination. This person assists in getting physician charts completed, pulls charts when necessary, and performs the regular medical records chart audit as opposed to the billing audit.

In addition to applying techniques to enable the hospital to produce a patient bill as soon after discharge as possible, it is also important to mail follow-up bills and to transfer unpaid accounts to the collection department on a timely basis. In many cases, if the hospital forgets the debtor, even for a short time, the debtor will forget the hospital. If the hospital has a monthly insurance trial balance by insurance company, a copy of this report should be mailed to each insurance company. Often the insurance company will investigate delinquent accounts.

Revenue foregone through the granting of cash discounts to either individuals or third party payers is not an allowable cost under current reimbursement schemes, even when it can be proven that overall savings would result. The hospital can grant cash discounts if, in the judgment of the chief financial officer, this would significantly speed up cash collections. However, these cash discounts cannot be reflected on the cost report. Another alternative is to charge interest for use of funds if the bill is more than 30 days delinquent, especially with third party payers. Few third party payers will pay interest on old accounts, and the hospital cannot legally force payment. However, stating an interest charge on the bill often speeds collections.

Many large third party payers will accept magnetic tape billing. If the hospital has electronic data-processing equipment, it should obtain permission to do tape billings with as many payers as possible. With tape billing, the hospital computer is programmed to produce a magnetic tape that is fed directly into the third party payer's computer. The hospital saves clerical expense, billing expense, and paper expense in addition to speeding up cash flow. The third party payer saves key punching expense. The most common tape billing arrangements are state Medicaid payments. Many states allow or encourage tape billing, especially from large hospitals. Problems with tape billing include difficulty in adapting to the very specific requirements of third party payers, adapting to changes in program requirements on very short notice, and rejected claims in large batch runs.

Billing Reports

Because of the importance to the hospital's financial stability, several weekly reports are customarily prepared to monitor this activity. In this section, several reports commonly used to monitor the billing function will be discussed.

The billing productivity report shows for each individual the amount of bills processed. An example of a billing productivity report for Community Hospital is shown in Table 4-1. This report can be prepared by type of account or in total. By using this report in conjunction with productivity standards, both supervisors and clerks know exactly what is expected of them and have a means of verifying that it is done. If used correctly, this report improves employee attitudes toward work because it shows that management is following their

Table 4–1 Community Hospital Billing Productivity Report

Week Ending June 15, 19XX

	Billable Accounts Invoiced			Nonbillable Accounts Resolved		
Employee	*Medicare*	*Medicaid*	*Other*	*Medicare*	*Medicaid*	*Other*
Smith	XX		X	X		
Jones		XX	X		X	
Drain			XX	X		X

performance with specific interest. The report also shows which employees are most productive. In using productivity reports, the hospital must monitor bills returned from third party payers to make sure employees are not producing unacceptable bills just to receive a high volume on the report.

Another useful tool is either a revenue-in-progress or billings-in-progress report. A revenue-in-progress report shows invoiced accounts pending payment while a billings-in-progress report shows only accounts that have not been invoiced. An example of a revenue-in-progress report for Community Hospital is shown in Table 4–2.

A large number of billable accounts not invoiced generally indicates a staffing problem. Billing backlog may be due to vacations, holidays, or unusually high census as well as to inadequate staffing. If the hospital knows it has good employees and the number of billable accounts not invoiced increases significantly, the staffing pattern should be reviewed.

Nonbillable accounts unresolved represents the most serious revenue-in-progress problem for most hospitals. The most common reasons for nonbillable accounts unresolved are:

- lack of a discharge diagnosis

- lack of insurance approval

Table 4–2 Community Hospital Revenue-In-Progress Report

Week Ending June 15, 19X0

	Type of Account			
Status	*Blue Cross*	*Medicare*	*Medicaid*	*Other*
Billable accounts not invoiced	XX	XX	XX	XX
Nonbillable accounts unresolved	XX	XX	XX	XX
Invoiced accounts pending payment	XXX	XXX	XXX	XXX

- lack of patient third party assignment
- denial of benefits pending receipt of more information.

Physicians who are delinquent in completing their charts at discharge present a problem common in some degree to all hospitals. Many physicians do not understand that the hospital cannot submit a bill until the chart is complete or do not understand the cash flow consequences of incomplete medical records' charts. Many hospitals suspend admitting privileges from physicians who are habitually behind in completing their charts.

The weekly revenue-in-progress report, productivity report, and all other billing reports should be circulated throughout the billing department. By keeping them informed of what is going on and why, the billing personnel are aware that they are an important part of the total patient care process.

BILLING PROCESS AND ACCOUNTING

In this section we will discuss several important functions and techniques to ensure that the billing functions are properly recorded in the hospital's general ledger.

Deductions from Revenue

The largest deductions from revenue in hospitals are contractual allowances. Contractual allowances represent a reduction from billed charges as a result of a contract between the hospital and a third party payer. The most common contractual allowances are Medicare, Medicaid, Blue Cross, county welfare, health maintenance organization agreements, and government social agency agreements.

Journal entries to record contractual allowances should be prepared by the billing personnel at the time of billing. Many hospitals post the allowance credit after payment is received instead of at the time of billing. This causes material distortions in monthly net revenue accounts as contractual allowances are shifted into the month of payment.

Other deductions should be carefully analyzed on a regular basis to determine whether they should continue to be shown as deductions from revenue or as expense items. If there is a possibility of being partially reimbursed from a cost-based payer, the amount should be shown as an expense item, not as a reduction of revenue. Examples of revenue deductions that have been reclassified to expense accounts by some hospitals include:

- bad debt expense that is allowable on some cost reports or rate review formulas

- Hill-Burton free care requirements that have been called interest expense because they represent a cost of obtaining funds

- employee and courtesy discounts that are allowable on some cost reports or rate review formulas.

The above examples are not all-inclusive. Each deduction from revenue should be aggressively studied to determine whether it is to the hospital's advantage to include it as an expense item. Reimbursement formulas and principles vary from state to state and often from county to county within a state.

General Ledger Controls

As we have noted, billing personnel should be responsible for processing journal entries to credit allowances, bad debt, and contractual adjustments in the month bills are processed. These entries must be carefully reviewed to make sure they are reasonable.

The accounts receivable amounts recorded on the balance sheet must equal the total of the individual balances. This is accomplished if the control accounts are posted automatically through the same process that is used to post charges as well as payments to the individual patient account. Once this is done, controls must be established to prevent changing totals except through the system. Often there is a tendency to attempt to short cut the system when posting a correction. Corrections should flow through the entire accounts receivable system.

It is important to balance in-house accounts to the applicable general ledger control accounts at the end of each month. This is especially critical if the hospital is not using electronic data-processing equipment.

CASHIERING

Cash is received by the hospital through the mail, over the cashier counter, from the cafeteria, from the parking garage, and from other sources.

Mail Receipts

All monies received by the hospital should be deposited daily. Most checks will be attached to a remittance advice or to an invoice. These should be applied to the proper account immediately. Other checks will be more difficult to apply and should be charged to a suspense account until the proper account can be identified. The balance in the suspense account should be carefully monitored. Often it takes several days to determine which account to charge monies received. It is easy to allow the balance in the unapplied cash or suspense account to get very large.

Two people should be present when the mail is opened. Checks should be stamped at once with a restrictive endorsement and all correspondence stapled to the check. An adding machine tape should be made of incoming mail. The total of the adding machine tape should be compared with the amount of the daily deposit.

The hospital can use a combined endorsement and data stamp. This stamp would include data needed to trace the accounts receivable posting directly from the cancelled check if a question should arise at a later date. An example of a combined endorsement and data stamp is:

Pay To the Order Of
First National Bank
For Deposit To Account 11–11000
Community Hospital
I.D. No. _____   Control No. _____
Account No. _____

Refunds

Patient refunds are growing problems for American hospitals. Definitive policies and procedures are needed to ensure that this function is carried out equitably. Patient refunds result when a bill is overpaid. The most common overpayment situation is a result of the patient having health care coverage from more than one insurance company. With the growing number of homes with two wage earners, many families are covered under two employer-paid group insurance plans. In addition, many Americans purchase supplemental insurance coverage to provide more protection than that offered under their primary health insurance policy. Overpayment can also result when a patient overpays the coinsurance or deductible portion of the hospital bill.

The first task in an overpayment situation is to search the accounts receivable records to determine whether or not the patient has another account with the hospital. This account could be for inpatient care under a prior admission, for outpatient care, or for care rendered to another family member. If there is a possibility that the patient had an account that was charged off, a search of prior bad debt expense should be made.

If there is any other account that a refund check can be applied to, the hospital should assume a right of offset. If the refund resulted because the patient paid part of the hospital bill, the funds can almost always be applied to another account. If the overpayment resulted because more than one insurance company paid for the hospital service, the hospital may be required to refund the overpayment to one of the insurance carriers.

After it has been determined that there is no other account and the overpayment must be refunded, the refund clerk must determine to whom the check should be sent. If two insurance companies have paid and there is a coordination-of-benefits clause that the hospital must comply with, the refund check must be sent to one of the insurance companies. Otherwise the refund check is sent to the patient. Every hospital should have well-defined refund policies that are rigidly adhered to.

Nonpatient Cashiering

Nonpatient cashiering includes such cash receipts as parking garage income, cafeteria receipts, pay telephone and vending machine commissions, student tuitions, silver recovery income, medical records transcription fees, and other miscellaneous income. Areas such as the parking garage, cafeteria, or coffee shop, and sometimes the gift shop, have full-time cashiers. Other cash receipts are handled by the same cashiers that process patient payments.

The hospital should have a daily cash report that summarizes cash receipts from all sources. This cash report is traced forward to the bank deposits and backward to the cash register tapes or other source documents. Because of the high exposure to fraud, cash must be carefully controlled. The best way to ensure against fraud is to have a highly regimented and detailed cash receipts system. The cashiering policies and procedures must be very narrowly defined, and most transactions should require that a form be filled out. Daily balancing functions should be on a standard form rather than on an adding machine tape or plain piece of paper.

SUMMARY

The billing and cashiering functions begin during the admitting or preadmitting process when information required to bill and to collect the account is obtained. All information contained on the admitting form must be verified as soon as possible.

Once the patient is admitted, it is important to minimize lost charges. The most effective way to accomplish this is to assign the head of each ancillary department the responsibility of managing, controlling, and maximizing that department's revenue and reducing its expenses. Hospital administration must support department head efforts by making sure that nurses, aides, clerks, orderlies, technicians, and other patient-care employees are properly trained and motivated to minimize lost charges. The cost of lost charges is directly proportional to the percentage of patients for which the hospital is reimbursed on the basis of billed charges. Reimbursement from cost-based payers, bad debts, and charity patients is generally not greatly affected by changes in the amount of lost charges or by price changes.

During the patient's hospital stay or outpatient visit, an estimate is made to determine the patient's liability. In order to accurately estimate this amount, the hospital must calculate the portion of the bill that will be paid by a third party payer or an agency and the portion that will be the responsibility of the patient. At discharge, the patient is asked to pay that estimated portion of the bill that is the patient's responsibility and is reminded that this estimate is tentative. The final bill must be prepared and sent to both third party payers and the patient in a timely manner. Follow-up bills on slow-pay accounts should be sent to insurance companies and other third party payers as aggressively as bills on self-pay accounts.

The billing function for most accounts begins with the appropriate billing screen. The billing screen is a prorated formula or process through which the hospital estimates the patient liability and the third party payer responsibility.

From the time of discharge to the time the first bill is sent, the account receivable is in the most crucial part of the billing process. To monitor this process, a series of billing reports is needed. A billing production report shows the number and/or amount of bills produced each week. This report is used in conjunction with productivity standards. Revenue-in-progress reports allow the hospital to monitor the status of unbilled accounts by type of payer.

The cashiering function should be controlled through very narrowly defined policies and procedures. Most hospitals utilize prenumbered forms, daily cash reports, cashier tie-out reports, and other forms to control the different aspects of the cash functions.

DISCUSSION QUESTIONS

1. Explain how the admitting department affects billing.
2. How can the hospital reduce the number of lost charges? How can the cash effect of lost charges be estimated?
3. Outline the steps in a hospital discharge procedure. In what ways does a good discharge procedure maximize hospital collections?
4. Explain what is meant by insurance screen or billing master.
5. What are some ways the hospital can shorten the billing lag?
6. What are the advantages of having weekly billing reports?
7. What are the most common reasons for nonbillable accounts that cannot be resolved? What can be done to eliminate these problems?
8. Explain how to set up a mail receipts procedure. What would you want to accomplish?
9. What are patient refunds?
10. How can the hospital ensure against fraud in cash receipt procedures?

Chapter 5

Credit and Collections

In the previous chapter we examined billing and cashiering as parts of accounts receivable management. In this chapter we discuss the credit and collection aspects of accounts receivable management.

The credit and collection function of a hospital cannot operate effectively unless administration has defined policies and procedures. These policies and procedures—or operating laws—of the credit and collection department involve a tradeoff between liquidity and public image. The operating laws needed to maximize liquidity will become clear in the following sections. The question of public image must be decided separately for each hospital. Once policies and procedures have been approved, administration has an obligation to defend credit personnel when complaints are made by patients, relatives, or other interested parties.

The first function of credit and collection is to determine who is responsible for payment. If a third party payer is responsible, the procedures are similar to those employed by commercial firms to collect trade accounts receivable. If an individual is responsible, the procedures are borrowed from commercial financial companies. Third party payer and self-pay receivables are reported, evaluated, and measured separately throughout the credit and collection function.

INITIAL PATIENT INFORMATION

Hospital patients are purchasing an unwanted service. Nobody wants to need the services of a modern hospital. The patients and their families are disturbed, emotionally upset, and often resent the hospital. Because the patient is a reluctant customer, it is important that the initial communication process set the proper tone in order for future collection efforts to be successful.

Information from the Patient

The responsibility to monitor information received from the patient is shared with the billing department. However, rejected bills, delinquent accounts, and bad debts reflect upon the results of credit and collections more than they do the billing department. Accurate and complete information from the patient is, therefore, more important to the credit department than it is to the billing department.

Most hospitals either require or encourage preadmitting forms from as many patients as possible. If preadmission information is collected, the patient's actual admission is made more smoothly and with a minimum of anxiety. The credit department is able to verify insurance coverage and estimate noncovered amounts. The credit history of self-pay patients can be investigated. If the hospital stay will impose a severe financial burden on the family, the attending physician can be contacted. Cash deposit requirements as well as other credit terms are easier to discuss over the telephone when the patient is in a familiar, secure environment than in the hospital at the time of admission.

The advantages of preadmission procedures are many. The most important impediment to a greater percentage of preadmissions is lack of cooperation from the admitting physician. Doctors do not object to preadmission forms; they are simply too busy to support and follow up on this practice.

Whether obtained prior to admission or at the time of admission, three types of information must be obtained from the patient: general information, third-party payer information, and credit information. General information needed by the credit and collections department includes name, address, telephone number, Social Security number, physician, dates of any prior admissions to the hospital, age, and information on the nearest relative. This information is required and monitored for completeness by other departments in the hospital.

Most patient accounts are covered, at least in part, by hospitalization insurance, Medicare, Medicaid, a health maintenance organization, or other third party payers. Because coverage is usually complex and difficult to determine, few patients have a good understanding of their hospitalization coverage. Therefore, all third party coverage must be verified as rapidly as possible. For Medicare, Blue Cross, and other large-volume payers the hospital will have a teletype or other efficient system. For other payers, either telephone or mail verification is necessary. Required information includes: name of payer, name of employer if applicable, group number, policy number, secondary coverage (i.e., major medical or coverage under spouse's insurance), limitations of coverage if known, coinsurance or deductible amounts, address and telephone number of payer, and dates of coverage. The patient should be asked if there is any other information that would help verify coverage from third party payers.

The third category of information that should be obtained for all patients is credit information. This information should include at least place of employment, current address as well as previous address, credit references, name of bank, and loans outstanding. Information on these points is needed to obtain a standard credit report.

Information to the Patient

An assignment-of-benefits form should be obtained for all possible third party coverage, and patients should be reminded that they are responsible for all amounts not covered by insurance. The hospital's credit policies should be explained in full. If a deposit is required, the patient or the patient's family must be told and the deposit collected. The discharge procedure as well as hospital policy covering billing before discharge should also be explained to the patient or family.

An estimate of the amount due from the patient should be made prior to admission. This gives the hospital some basis on which to establish a projected payment plan.

THIRD PARTY PAYER RECEIVABLES

From 75 to 90 percent of hospital receivables are due from third party payers. These include Medicare, Medicaid, Blue Cross, other commercial insurance companies, health maintenance organizations, workmen compensation claims, and other government or agency receivables.

Cost of Lending to Third Party Payers

Generally, a hospital can assume that verified third party payer claims will not be charged off as bad debts. However, collection efforts are required to decrease the collection time between billing and receipt of cash. Third party receivables represent the extension of open-account credit by the hospital to the company or agency responsible for payment. These obligations represent an important source of interest-free borrowings for most insurance companies and government agencies. A hospital that does not closely monitor and use collection techniques will find their investment in receivables becoming greater as the collection time becomes longer.

The interest cost to the hospital of investment in receivables is easy to determine. The cost is calculated by multiplying the average annual investment in receivables by the highest interest rate being paid on long-term debt. If the receivables exceed total long-term debt, the excess receivables are multiplied by the average interest rate the hospital could earn on short-term investments.

To illustrate this calculation, assume a hospital has twenty million dollars in accounts receivable and fifteen million dollars in long-term debt. The hospital is paying nine percent interest on its long-term debt and could earn six percent interest on temporary investments. The cost to the hospital of investment in receivables is:

$$\$15,000,000 \times .09 = \$1,340,000$$
$$\$5,000,000 \times .06 = \underline{300,000}$$

Total Annual Interest Cost $1,640,000

Because of its investment in receivables, the hospital in this example has $1,640,000 less cash to spend on equipment, to pay employee salaries, or to provide additional services. To the payer the savings from withholding payment is substantial. A government agency that borrows funds at an interest rate of seven percent can save seven million dollars per year by increasing the average amount due hospitals by one hundred million dollars. For both sides the interest involved is substantial.

In addition to the interest cost of receivables, the hospital absorbs collection costs to collect these receivables. To calculate collection cost, the average number of full-time equivalent personnel (including an estimate for supervision) that work on third party payer receivables is multiplied by the average annual salary. Then a percent for fringe benefits and an estimate of nonsalary cost are added. To illustrate, assume the hospital has five full-time equivalent personnel that verify coverage, file, and follow up on third party payer accounts. Their average salary is $10,000 per year. Cash fringe benefits for the hospital approximate 20 percent of salary expense, and the credit manager estimates that 70 percent of the $10,000 nonsalary cost budgeted for the credit department will be for third party accounts. Total collection cost for the hospital is:

Salary expense 5 @ $10,000	$50,000
Fringe benefits @ 20%	10,000
Nonsalary expense	7,000
Total collection cost	$67,000

The hospital also experiences an opportunity cost if a wanted expenditure was turned down because funds were not available from lenders, endowment funds, or other sources. This opportunity cost is equal to the additional net gain that would have been generated if this expenditure had been made. The net gain could be from additional revenue or from decreased expenses. Calculation of opportunity costs for a nonprofit community hospital is not within the scope of this book.

Thus, the total known cost of twenty million dollars in third party payer receivables for the hospital in our example is:

Interest cost	$1,640,000
Collection cost	67,000
Total	$1,707,000

Reducing Third Party Receivables

We have defined third party receivables as the extension of open-account credit by the hospital to the company or agency responsible for payment. This definition represents the key to credit and collection procedures used to reduce these receivables. Hospitals should follow the same procedures major corporations follow to reduce their trade receivables.

Constant pressure must be exerted at all times on third party payers. Earlier in this chapter we saw how hospital payables are an important, as well as valuable, source of financing. No motivation exists to voluntarily pay hospitals in a shorter time period. Rather, the motivation is to lengthen the pay period—an action that increases hospital receivables.

Dunning is one of the most commonly used collection tools because it is a relatively inexpensive and simple technique. Hospitals have an enviable opportunity when using this technique. When reminders are sent to insurance companies or governmental agencies, reminders should also be sent to the patients. This tells them that their bills have not been paid and also that the ultimate responsibility for payment rests with them. Often this is the most effective collection technique, especially with governmental agencies.

Telephone calls should be made to follow up on past due accounts. If a hospital has been experiencing many problems with a particular payer, a personal call should be made to the claims manager. If all else fails, legal action should be initiated. Often legal collection procedures are settled before the court date. In this case, the legal procedure acts as a catalyst to solve the problem.

Commercial insurance companies, health maintenance organizations, and others depend on trade credit. If the hospital believes a company is a slow payer, that fact should be reported to the commercial credit agencies. This is the standard procedure to follow in our commercial system. In addition, there is an incentive to reduce outstanding payables to a particular hospital if this will clear up a poor credit reputation.

Government agencies normally attach little importance to commercial credit report histories. An effective way to reduce government receivables is through the political process. Legislatures are usually eager to protect hospitals from the bureaucrats but they must be armed with facts. State and national hospital associations are often helpful in organizing, as well as summarizing, information from large numbers of hospitals.

SELF-PAY RECEIVABLES

Although self-pay represents a small portion of total hospital receivables, it is the source of nearly all bad-debt losses. In order to keep bad debts at a minimum, self-pay receivables often receive a disproportionate amount of credit and collection effort. The calculation of collection cost and interest cost due to holding self-pay receivables is identical to the process explained in the section on third party receivables. In this section we will discuss the techniques for reducing self-pay receivables as well as minimizing bad-debt losses.

Attempts To Shift the Costs

We have seen that the costs of holding accounts receivable are very high. With self-pay receivables the hospital often has an opportunity to shift these costs to banks, finance companies, or credit card companies. These companies are specialists in consumer lending, are efficient, and make a substantial profit. Often it is advantageous to both the hospital and the consumer lending company if the costs can be shifted. Whenever possible, the hospital should make every attempt to shift the costs.

Accepting credit cards represents one of the easiest ways to eliminate patient receivables. Visa, Mastercard, American Express, Diners, Carte Blanche, and many other credit card companies can be considered. Credit cards are especially suitable for outpatients and for small balances of noncovered inpatient bills. For inpatients who have no third party coverage or very limited coverage, the amount is usually too large for credit card financing. If the hospital accepts cards, there will be a discount charged by the credit card company. The amount of the discount depends upon the company, the dollar volume, and other factors determined by the credit card company. If the discount is three percent, the hospital will receive $97 in cash for every $100 in receivables turned over. The discount should be recorded as an expense rather than a deduction from revenue. Both accounting treatments are acceptable. However, treating these discounts as an expense is the only way to get reimbursed from third party cost payers (i.e., Medicare, Medicaid, and others).

Another way to attempt to shift the cost of holding these receivables is to arrange a direct loan to the patient from a bank or finance company. There are many different kinds of direct-loan arrangements the hospital can negotiate. The most common are: with recourse, with a guarantee, a discounted note, and a direct no-recourse note. With recourse is the least desirable of these alternatives, and a direct no-recourse note is the most desirable. The reason for this ranking will become clear as we define what these terms mean.

With recourse in effect means that the hospital is a cosigner on the note. (The patient should never be made aware of this fact because it makes future collection efforts less effective.) The patient signs a note payable to the bank or finance company, and the hospital signs a recourse agreement on the back of the note. The recourse agreement makes the hospital equally and jointly responsible. Only routine collection efforts will be made, and, if the note becomes three or four months past due, the hospital will have to pay the note off in full with interest and often late charges. The only advantage of this kind of financing is the fact that it is easy to obtain, especially if the patient has a very poor credit record. The patient often pays the note off in full, and even when they do default, it is usually after at least some installments have been paid.

A note that the hospital guarantees, either in full or up to a stated dollar amount, is much more desirable than one with recourse. A guarantee obligates the hospital to pay the bank or finance company only after all normal collection efforts, including legal action, have been exhausted. Lenders must exert more aggressive collection efforts at their cost before they look to the hospital for payment.

A discounted note relieves the hospital of all future liability to the lender. The lender negotiates a discount amount with the hospital after both have had a chance to study a credit report on the patient. Depending on the creditworthiness of the patient, as well as the credit policy of the lending institution, this discount could be very substantial. Unlike the discount on credit cards, a discount on notes is not recognized as a normal collection expense by most cost payers. Rather, it is treated as a deduction from revenue and absorbed 100 percent by the hospital.

A direct no-recourse note is a direct loan by the lender to the patient to pay the hospital bill. The hospital handles all of the paper work for the lender but has no future liability and receives full payment for the billed charges. If the patient has a good credit record, is employed, and the bill is within the patient's ability to repay, the hospital should not accept one of the less desirable financing mechanisms without a great deal of resistance.

When negotiating financing arrangements, the hospital should keep in mind that the bank or financing company will make a healthy profit on the business. The arrangement will be mutually beneficial, and the hospital has a great deal of bargaining leverage. If satisfactory terms cannot be negotiated, a hospital or group of hospitals should consider organizing a captive finance company that deals exclusively with health care receivables. The services of a captive finance company could also be offered to the medical staff and other health care providers.

Free care is another mechanism that can be used to shift the cost of carrying receivables. The most obvious free-care arrangements are through a government or charitable agency. The credit department should work very closely with the hospital's own social service department as well as with state and county social workers. In addition, most hospitals have received Hill-Burton or other government funds in the past that have a free-care requirement. Until the hospital has met its mandated free-care requirement for the year, any accounts charged to free care are a shift of accounts receivable costs. Of course, if the free-care requirement has already been met, there is only a conceptual difference between free care and bad debts.

Self-Pay Collections

When the patient was admitted, every attempt was made to receive accurate information. Third party payer resources were exhausted, the hospital's credit and collection policies were fully explained to the patient, an attempt was made to collect a cash deposit, and a major effort was made to shift the cost of holding accounts receivable. All of the above were attempts to minimize the self-pay receivables. The hospital is now confronted with trying to minimize its losses on this most expensive classification of receivables. It is not unusual for losses on the accounts remaining in this category to exceed 50 percent. Most of the techniques for dealing with self-pay accounts are well known and need only be mentioned here.

Dun letters are the easiest and cheapest way to effect mass collections. These letters should be planned so they become increasingly more persuasive. The timing of the letters should be systematic. At some point, the form letters should be replaced with either a telephone call or a personally written letter. Many habitually poor payers do not believe an account is serious enough to worry about until they receive a telephone call or a personal letter. Since the hospital is competing with other creditors for funds, they cannot rely solely on form letters.

If extensive telephone collections are made, the hospital should hire personnel to do this on the evening shift. Telephone collections are much more efficient in the evening because more people are at home at that time.

Throughout the collection process, timely followup is important. A good system of identifying and performing additional collection efforts in a carefully timed sequence is essential.

Finally, it is important to remember that patients are admitted and new accounts receivable are generated every month. Many hospitals are caught in the trap of spending too much effort on delinquent self-pay accounts while the millions of dollars tied up in third party receivables continue to grow. It should be a hospital policy to turn accounts regularly over to commercial collection agencies.

Collection agencies normally retain a predetermined percentage of accounts collected. This percentage is negotiated. When dealing with collection agencies, the hospital should keep in mind that the agency will make a profit when accounts are assigned to them. The arrangement is mutually beneficial, and the hospital has negotiating leverage.

CREDIT AND COLLECTION COST RETURN

The actual amount of money that a hospital should spend on credit and collection efforts cannot be precisely determined. In each case, the amount will depend on some empirical assumptions. These assumptions can be determined only by examining the costs of holding accounts receivable at a given level and assuming the incremental change in costs that would result at a different level. Alternative costs at both higher and lower levels of accounts receivable should be examined.

Earlier in this chapter we saw how to calculate the cost of carrying third party receivables. The total cost was the sum of interest costs plus collection costs. This is represented by the following formula:

$$TC = (I \times AR) + CC$$

where:

TC = total costs
I = average interest rate
AR = accounts receivable
CC = collection costs

As we increase collection costs, accounts receivable will decrease, thereby reducing holding costs. To minimize collection costs, we need to examine several alternatives using empirical judgment to determine the effect on accounts receivable. Our formula now becomes:

$$TC = I (AR \pm \Delta AR) + CC \pm \Delta CC$$

where:

TC = total costs
I = average interest rate
AR = accounts receivable
ΔAR = change in accounts receivable
CC = collection costs
ΔCC = change in collection costs

The cost of carrying self-pay receivables is identical to the cost of holding third party receivables except we now need to consider bad-debt losses. As collection costs are increased, both interest costs and bad-debt costs will decrease. The formula is:

$$TC = (I \times AR) = BD + CC$$

where:

TC = total costs
I = average interest rate
AR = accounts receivable
BD = bad-debt losses
CC = collection costs

Using empirical judgment, we can minimize total costs of holding self-pay receivables by applying the following formula:

where:
$$TC = I (AR \pm \Delta AR) + (BD \pm \Delta BD) + (CC \pm \Delta CC)$$

TC = total costs
I = average interest rate
AR = accounts receivable
ΔAR = change in accounts receivable
BD = bad-debt losses
ΔBD = change in bad-debt losses
CC = collection costs
ΔCC = change in collection costs

By examining these two equations together we can calculate whether additional collection costs should be added to the third party payer receivables or the self-pay receivables. We can also calculate whether collection effort should be shifted from one type of receivable to the other. By calculating the costs separately, we are able to both minimize total collection costs and maximize our return from collection efforts.

EVALUATION OF CREDIT OPERATIONS

Because much of the work of the credit and collection department involves sensitive interpersonal relationships with patients, it is very difficult to evaluate the work of this department objectively. Depending on whether one hears stories told by the credit and collection personnel or stories told by disgruntled patients, the personnel in the credit and collection department are either effective workers or heartless people. It is extremely difficult to make a fair, objective judgment concerning this department without meaningful objective facts.

Interpersonal relationships with patients or with third party payers should be evaluated against established policies and procedures that have been defined or approved by administration. Without these policies and procedures, or operating laws, the credit and collection department cannot be effective. These policies and procedures should be reviewed regularly to ascertain whether or not they are still valid. Exceptions to them should be approved by administration on a case-by-case basis.

In addition to evaluating compliance with policies and procedures, it is necessary to determine whether the credit and collection department is effective in minimizing the cost of carrying accounts receivable. Several forms of analysis can be employed.

Accounts Receivable Reports

We noted earlier that third party payer receivables and self-pay receivables should be evaluated separately. Table 5–1 shows the basic aging of an accounts

Table 5-1 Community Hospital—Comparative Aging of Accounts

As of June 30, 19X1
in Thousands

Days delinquent:	Total	Current	30–60	60–90	90–180	180–260	Over 360
Blue Cross	$10,800	$ 6,480	$3,240	$ 540	$ 400	$ 120	$ 20
Medicare	6,000	4,100	1,120	600	60	30	90
Medicaid	1,200	120	135	400	480	35	30
Commercial insurance	1,500	900	400	100	25	50	25
Other third party	500	90	100	85	100	100	25
Total third party	20,000	11,690	4,995	1,725	1,065	335	190
Self-pay	4,000	200	210	590	900	1,000	1,100
Total receivables	$24,000	$11,890	$5,205	$2,315	$1,965	$1,335	$1,290
Percent of total analysis:							
Third party	100.0	58.4	25.0	8.6	5.3	1.7	1.0
Self-pay	100.0	5.0	5.2	14.8	22.5	25.0	27.5
Total receivables	100.0	49.5	21.7	9.6	8.2	5.6	5.4

receivable report. This report shows an aging of each major third party payer receivable. After analyzing the report, it is easy to identify where the major problems lie. The report shows total third party, as well as self-pay receivables, by age in both dollars and percent.

Comparative Analysis

The basic aging of accounts receivable by type of payer is useful in judging data of a single period. However, the data become much more useful when compared with other data.

The most common comparative reports show the current period with prior-year receivables. This does not adjust the figures for revenue yield per adjusted patient day, however, and may be misleading (see Chapter 7 for a discussion of revenue yield per adjusted patient day). Revenue per adjusted patient day increases every year for inflation, utilization, and intensity. One could mentally adjust comparative figures for inflation. However, utilization and intensity are too complicated to adjust mentally. Only gross approximations of performance can be made from agings of unadjusted comparative accounts receivables.

The actual data can also be compared with a budgeted or forecasted figure. It is more desirable to compare an aging of accounts receivable report with an industry norm or area average if available. However, in most regions norms and averages are not available in enough detail to be useful.

Percentage Analysis

In Table 5–2, the amount as well as the percentage change in each item is compared. Percentage analysis can be calculated by payer, by age of accounts, or in total.

The comparative analysis is very useful to indicate trends within the aging categories. However, this analysis does not adjust accounts receivable for inflation, utilization, and intensity. There is a strong temptation to examine an individual line item without recognizing these three complex factors.

Vertical percentage analysis is a useful method of showing the composition of accounts receivable as well as the changes in total accounts receivable. An example of vertical percentage analysis is shown in Table 5–3.

Table 5–3 is an excellent tool to help plan where to place the greatest collection emphasis. If calculated on a monthly basis, this analysis can assist the credit manager in planning short-term collection strategy.

Common Size Analysis

The most accurate analysis of accounts receivable is made through common size analysis. In a common size analysis all figures are converted to a common

Table 5–2 Community Hospital—Comparative Accounts Receivable Aging

June 30, 19X0 and 19X1
in Thousands

Age	Total June 30, 19X0	Total June 30, 19X1	Increases (Decreases) Amount	Increases (Decreases) Percent
Current	$10,280	$11,890	$1,610	15.7
30–60	5,010	5,205	195	3.9
60–90	1,115	2,315	1,200	107.6
90–180	1,570	1,965	395	25.1
180–360	1,110	1,335	225	20.3
Over 360	1,075	1,290	215	20.0
Total	$20,160	$24,000	$3,840	19.0

Table 5–3 Community Hospital—Percentage Analysis of Accounts Receivable

June 30, 19X0 and 19X1
in Thousands

	19X0	19X1	Percentages 19X0	Percentages 19X1
Blue Cross	$ 8,680	$10,800	43.1	45.0
Medicare	4,940	6,000	24.5	25.0
Medicaid	1,010	1,200	5.0	5.0
Commercial insurance	1,480	1,500	7.3	6.2
Other third party	400	500	2.0	2.1
Total third party	16,510	20,000	81.9	83.3
Self-pay	3,650	4,000	18.1	16.7
Total receivables	$20,160	$24,000	100.0	100.0

size base. A good base to use is number of days revenue in accounts receivable. The following formula can be used to calculate the number of days revenue in accounts receivable.

$$\text{Days revenue} = \frac{\text{A/R} \times 365}{\text{Patient revenue}}$$

where:

Days revenue = number of days of average patient revenue represented by the category of accounts receivable being studied

A/R = dollar value of net accounts receivable in the category being studied

Patient revenue = projected or budgeted patient revenue for the current year and actual patient revenue for prior years

The number of days revenue in accounts receivable is sometimes referred to as the average collection period. If the hospital has a computer, comparative statements expressed in number of days revenue or average collection period can be routinely prepared. If these statements cannot be prepared automatically, it is a simple task for a clerk to prepare this comparison manually each month.

Indexing represents another form of common size analysis. Indexing is used extensively by the U.S. government in reporting the Consumer Price Index, labor statistics, and many other analyses. To use indexing, the hospital defines the average revenue per adjusted patient day in the base year as 100. Average revenue per adjusted patient day in subsequent years is then compared to the base year to compute an appropriate deflation. This deflation can be used to convert accounts-receivable aging reports into base-year dollars.

Whatever method of converting is employed by the hospital, it is important to remember the purpose of common size analysis. The purpose is to adjust comparative years simultaneously for differences in (1) prices, (2) intensity, and (3) utilization of ancillaries.

The comparative analyses illustrated in this chapter do not by themselves identify credit and collection department performance. They only help identify where potential strengths and weaknesses lie and suggest areas of investigation that may lead to improved results.

SUMMARY

The credit and collection function of a hospital cannot operate effectively unless administration has defined policies and procedures. Throughout the administration of these policies, it is important to keep in mind two fundamental principles: (1) hospital patients are purchasing an unwanted service, and (2) it is to the advantage of third party payers to delay payment to the hospital as long as possible. Therefore, the basic tasks are to motivate self-pay patients to pay and to reduce the collection lag for third party payers.

The greatest cost of accounts receivable is related to the time value of money. This can be called the interest cost of holding accounts receivable. In addition to the interest cost of receivables, the hospital absorbs collection costs to maintain these receivables, and the hospital assumes an opportunity cost equal to the net gain that would have resulted if the hospital had cash rather than receivables.

Because third party receivables represent the extension of credit by the hospital to the agency responsible for payment, the hospital must be aggressive in these collection efforts. Self-pay receivables represent a small portion of total hospital receivables. However, self-pay receivables are the source of nearly all bad-debt losses.

DISCUSSION QUESTIONS

1. Why is it important to receive accurate information from the patient during the admission process?
2. Discuss the three types of information that are obtained from the patient during the admitting process.
3. How would you calculate the interest cost of patient accounts receivable?
4. Define lost opportunity cost of holding patient accounts receivable.
5. What are some of the techniques that can be used to shift the cost of holding self-pay receivables?
6. How can the hospital evaluate whether it should expend more effort on self-pay receivables or on third party payer receivables if there are only enough funds to do one of these?
7. Explain the difference between a comparative analysis and a common size analysis.

Chapter 6

Budgeting Expenses

In this chapter we will discuss the hospital's comprehensive plan that quantifies goals in terms of specific financial and operating objectives. We will also examine the need for a budget, some techniques, and the budget process.

NEED FOR A BUDGET

In this section we will discuss the need for a budget from a logical point of view. We will then examine the human reasons and the business reasons for a comprehensive hospital budget.

Budget Evolution

Each of us makes budget decisions constantly throughout the day. We go to the grocery store and make a decision to buy ground beef rather than steak, even though we prefer steak and have enough money to purchase it. We visit a new car showroom and must choose between a large automobile and a small automobile. We use a piece of scratch paper to calculate our cash available and make a choice that is at least somewhat less than optimum. In purchasing a new home, we calculate present earnings, expected future earnings, sacrifices we are willing to make, and other factors. The decision of how much to spend on a home takes several hours or several days and involves an organized process.

In each of the above decisions we had to make a choice because of limited funds. As the decision-making process became more difficult we started to formalize the process in order to reduce the risk. Most of our personal decisions are relatively simple, and we do not need a formal process.

Let us extend this budget process analysis to the business environment. For people who sell Avon cosmetics part-time out of their homes, most decisions are made without a formal budget process. An entrepreneur in a neighborhood grocery, however, will sit down regularly to calculate budget goals and set objectives. If the business grows to a chain of several supermarkets, a well defined process is needed to make sure all elements important to the decision process are combined. The manager of each store will submit plans for that store, and all such plans will be negotiated at the central office. It would be foolish for the head of a chain of supermarkets to make a budget without involving the store managers because the business is so complex that no one person can remember all the important details.

The point is that as business entities become more complex, the budget process becomes more complex and more people must become involved.

Hospital budget decisions are not unlike the decisions made by individuals or by grocery stores. As hospitals become larger and more complex, it becomes important to have a plan that involves department heads in a well-defined process. Large medical centers require a more complicated budget process than a 50-bed rural hospital does. However, it should be noted that all hospitals today are complex entities as well as big-business enterprises. No hospital can have a workable budget without department-head involvement in a well-defined process.

Human Aspects of Budgeting

In spite of the existence of computers and automation, people still operate hospitals. Employees do not like to fumble along from day to day not knowing the game plan and without being involved in the decision-making process. They want to be involved in managing their departments, and want to know the goals and objectives of the hospital. Because of this, the human aspects of budgeting are much more important than accounting techniques.

For a budget to be most effective, the concept must have the full backing of the administrator. A skeptical top-management attitude will trickle down to the detriment of the entire hospital. Strong administrative support will also trickle down to the rest of the hospital.

In addition to obtaining administrative support, it is important to remember that a budget is a central tool that places the manager in the spotlight. The natural reaction to restriction and control is resistance and self-defense. Ideally, hospital personnel should view the budget as a positive tool by which their department can be improved. The budget should not be regarded as a heinous type of management pressure. However, to avoid this requires management selling and education. It also requires participatory budgeting. A weak budget developed from the bottom up is a better control tool than a strong budget developed from the top down.

If the department managers develop and negotiate their own budget, the natural human tendencies of resistance and self-defense work for the hospital rather than against the hospital. If the department heads view the budget as their own plan, then in self-defense they will fight to make it work and will resist anything that causes significant budget variances.

It cannot be overemphasized that a healthy acceptance of the budget is very difficult to achieve in a hospital. Partial success takes a minimum of two years after participatory budgeting is initiated, and total success is probably non-existent.

Business Aspects of Budgeting

The business objectives of a budget program are to:

- provide a written expression of the plans of the hospital in quantitative terms
- provide a basis for the evaluation of financial performance in accordance with the plans
- provide a useful tool for the control of costs
- create cost awareness throughout the hospital.

In other words, budgeting is simply compelled and quantified planning. It is the planning and controlling of a business in an organized, methodical manner. A budget process produces financial proforma statements that show what the results will be if present plans are implemented. If the results are not acceptable, there is still time to change the plan. There is no need for a hospital to drift along until it is caught in an undesirable situation that should have been anticipated and avoided.

THE BUDGET PROCESS

In this section we will go through the budget process. The principles outlined in this process should be followed by all American hospitals.

Budget Calendar

The first document in the hospital's budget process is the budget calendar. This lists the dates of each segment of the budget process, tells who is responsible for the segment, and provides a brief narrative to explain the purpose of the segment and to show how it fits into the total budget process.

The purpose of the budget calendar is to make a plan for the completion of the budget in time to meet outside constraints and to set deadlines. All personnel who have a role in the annual budget should see the entire plan so that they know how their part fits into the overall plan. They should see how missing a deadline will affect others and should know about deadlines imposed by others.

To make up a budget calendar, the first task is to list each step in the budget process, highlighting those that either are imposed by others or for some reason are inflexible. The budget process includes the following steps:

- Prepare statistical assumptions, including, but not limited to, patient days by service, changes in building gross square feet, introduction of new services and projected dates, number of procedures for the major departments (laboratory, radiology, and so on), and number of outpatient visits.

- Prepare economic forecasts that include salary inflation factors; fringe-benefit inflation factors; inflation factors for supplies and other nonsalary items detailed by major expense item and by department; new developments that may affect the hospital, such as additional physicians joining the staff, physicians leaving the staff, additions to other hospitals in the service area, or major clinics under construction; proposed legislation or government regulations, if they are expected to pass or be implemented; and any other factor that might affect the hospital's income or expense during the budget period.

- Distribute budget packages to department heads. These packages will include assumptions, forms, schedules, and historical data for each department. It is best to distribute the packages at a department head meeting and to have at least one hour of formal instruction in budget techniques and accounting constraints.

- Give technical assistance to department heads as they prepare the first drafts of their budget requests. Prepare budget goals and policies for the period. These will constitute an outline of the financial plan. They may include a targeted net gain or loss, a marketing strategy, third party payer strategy, or any other item that has a bearing upon the hospital's finances.

- Obtain approval of budget assumptions, goals, and policies. Depending upon the hospital, this may mean governing board approval, approval by a committee of the governing board, administrative approval, or operating budget committee approval.

- Hold departmental budget hearings. Those present should include the controller, the administrator or assistant administrator, and the department head. It is also a good idea to attempt to have a board member present during each budget hearing. This makes the department heads feel they have been heard and at the same time provides board members with an excellent opportunity to learn the intricacies of day-to-day hospital operating problems.

- Prepare typed summaries of each budget hearing. This documents promises and statements made between administration and department heads. These summaries will be referred to throughout the year as budget variances are investigated. If the typed summaries include personal observations and impressions of the controller, they should be shared only with administration. If these summaries are rather formal and include only factual information, a copy of each summary can be given to the appropriate department head. The format and distribution of budget hearing summaries will depend upon the preferences of the controller and the administrator.

- Summarize the individual department budgets into a first draft of the master budget. After reviewing this for reasonableness, the controller's department summarizes the total budget into a format to be presented to the board or a committee of the board. This presentation will be enhanced by graphs, descriptive narrative, and comparative historical data.

After making revisions mandated by the governing board, the budget is submitted to any relevant outside agency for approval. Many states have a formal rate review process. Others have a required rate and budget review process by a major third party payer. In addition, Medicare intermediaries require a review of the budget and proposed rates before the start of the fiscal year.

After approval by outside agencies, each department should be given a detailed copy of its approved budget for the period. At the same time, many hospitals take this opportunity to hold a news conference in which the local press is given highlights of the approved budget. With proper planning, this can be used to gain public support for the hospital's objectives. The press conference can be prepared with the help of an outside consultant.

The above example of functions that can be included in the budget calendar is not all-inclusive, nor will the functions described be applicable to all hospitals. Each hospital must examine its own budget process in developing the list of functions to be included in the published budget calendar. It is better to list too many functions than to provide inadequate detail. After the functions have been developed, the controller must assign a due date and identify the person or persons responsible. The budget calendar is then distributed to all departments.

Budget Assumptions

In some hospitals, information on projected patient statistics, additional services, proposed salary increases, economic factors, hospital goals, expense policies, and other pertinent information never reaches the department heads. This is because the information is rationed rather than shared, with each department head's ration being only that information that appears to affect that department directly. This approach fails to take into account the complexity and intricate interrelationships that exist. If the operating room will do 25 percent more procedures next year, this will have a ripple effect on nursing service, laundry, linen, central supply, pharmacy, lab, anesthesiology, maintenance, housekeeping, and many other departments. Other budget assumptions will have a similar ripple effect on other hospital departments.

The major purpose of budget assumptions is to share as much information as possible with all departments. That way the entire hospital will be planning on the same track. A group cohesiveness is created, and the budget variances throughout the year will be easier to explain.

Budget assumptions should also be used as a tool to initiate cost-containment measures and to announce any new policy that directly affects expenses in either a positive or negative manner. Assumptions set the tone of the budget. The hospital may want to increase expenses in order to increase the quality of care or patient convenience. On the other hand, the hospital may want to reduce significantly the rate of increase in costs per patient day. The important point is that through budget assumptions the hospital has a choice and can directly influence the result.

Exhibit 6–1 is an abbreviated list of assumptions for Community Hospital.

An average community hospital should have a minimum of 25 assumptions, and a major medical center may have as many as 100 assumptions.

Nonsalary Worksheet

The nonsalary worksheets contain historical data that are used by department heads in conjunction with the budget assumptions to prepare an estimate of

---

Exhibit 6–1 Community Hospital Budget Assumptions

Fiscal Year Ended June 30, 19X0

1. All approved budgets are subject to the availability of funds.
2. A CT body scanner will be operational in September.
3. Two family practice physicians, one pediatrician, one nephrologist, and up to four other physicians will be added to the active staff in the first six months of the year.
4. Supply costs will increase as follows: drugs six percent, medical supplies eight percent, chemicals nine percent, services eight percent, food nine percent.
5. Reimbursement for use of an employee's personal automobile will be increased from $.16 per mile to $.19 per mile.
6. Patient days will increase approximately five percent over last year.

nonsalary expense requirements for the budget period. An example of a nonsalary worksheet is shown in Exhibit 6–2.

Hospital department heads normally have some difficulty using account numbers properly. Therefore, the budget worksheet package should have a glossary

Exhibit 6–2 Community Hospital Nonsalary Expense Worksheet

19X0 Budget Preparation

Department: _____

Account	Account Description	Actual 6 mo.		Budget Request	
		19X8	*19X9*	*19X9*	*19X0*
200	Central service				
300	Supplies, nonpatient				
305	Supplies, patient				
310	Drugs				
500	Small equipment				
600	Travel & education				
700	Repairs & service				
TOTALS					

of terms attached. At the department head meeting when the budget packages are distributed, the controller should be prepared to explain the hospital's chart of accounts. In addition, half-day seminars should be given periodically by the business office to acquaint newly hired clerks, secretaries, nurses, department heads, and others with the travel policy, accounting approval policies, payroll procedures, unique forms, and an in-depth study of the chart of accounts. Because the hospital's chart of accounts is the focal point of the general ledger and of accounting reports, it is important that every person in the hospital understand how to use it properly.

The historical information provided should include at least one full year's actual expense, the current year's budget, and a portion of the current year's actual. The number of months included in the current year's actual should always be a number that can be mentally annualized. For example, if at the time the budget package is prepared the hospital has seven months of actual experience, the worksheets should include only six months of actual. If the hospital has five months of actual experience when the budget packages are prepared, the worksheets should include four months of actual for the current year. This is because six months can be doubled mentally, while a seven-month data period will only confuse the department head. Four months of data can easily be tripled, but a five-month data period is meaningless in the preparation of an annual request.

The individual department heads now have a budget calendar to establish due dates, a set of budget assumptions to set the tone of hospital spending and to establish parameters, and several columns of historical data detailed by account for each department. Armed with this information, most managers will have no difficulty preparing a budget request. A few, however, will need technical assistance from the controller's office.

Personnel Requirements Worksheet

Personnel costs in a hospital cannot be effectively budgeted or controlled without some type of formal position control system. A position control system is sometimes confused with the employee master list, which is a personnel department control tool. The position control is a budget and expense control tool. It itemizes by department all approved positions by shift and by job title. When an employee terminates, no change is made in the position control. The department head simply has a vacant approved position that can be filled. When employees are hired, they are slotted into an approved position. Administrative control is exercised over positions. Department control is exercised over employees assigned to approved positions. A sample position control for the radiology department is shown in Table 6–1 below.

The personnel requirements worksheet should be used only to request changes in the present position control. This includes planned reductions, requested additions, and planned changes in job descriptions, such as replacing registered

Table 6–1 Community Hospital Position Control

Department: 603 — Radiology

Pos. No.	Biwkly Hours	Job Title	Hourly Pay Rate Level			
			1	2	3	4
712.1	80	Manager of radiology	Salary Payroll			
712.2	80	Spec procedure tech	5.50	5.75	6.00	6.25
712.3	80	Senior technologist	5.50	5.75	6.00	6.25
712.4	80	Registered technologist	4.75	5.00	5.25	5.50
712.5	80	Registered technologist	4.75	5.00	5.25	5.50
712.6	80	Registered tech — nights	5.00	5.25	5.50	5.75
712.7	32	Registered tech	4.75	5.00	5.25	5.50
712.8	32	Registered tech	4.75	5.00	5.25	5.50
712.9	32	Registered tech — nights	5.00	5.25	5.50	5.75
712.10	80	Medical transcriber	4.50	4.75	5.00	5.25
712.11	80	Film librarian	4.25	4.50	4.75	5.00
712.12	80	Radiology clerk	4.00	4.25	4.50	4.75
712.13	56	RT on call	1.00	1.00	1.00	1.00
	872	Total budgeted hours				

nurses with licensed practical nurses or replacing a secretary with a clerk typist. It should be understood by department managers that if a completed worksheet is not received, it will be assumed that the present department manpower is satisfactory.

Predictably, it will be necessary to deny many requests for additional personnel each year because of limited funds and cost-containment pressures. Therefore, the personnel requirements worksheet should contain enough information to enable administration to make an informed decision. Exhibit 6–3 is an example of a personnel requirements worksheet for Community Hospital.

On Exhibit 6–3 worksheet, it is assumed that the hospital has a biweekly pay period. Biweekly hours requested should not exceed one full-time equivalent, which is 80 hours. If the position must be staffed seven days per week, a request for a full-time position should be submitted for five days and a request for a part-time position should be submitted for the remaining two days.

After changes in the position control are approved, the controller's department calculates budgeted salary expense by department. This calculation takes into account the cost-of-living pay increases, approved changes in the position control, the effect of any applicable union contracts, and other information that would not be available to department heads when their budgets were prepared. This calculation should consider the effect of vacation coverage, overtime pay, shift differential, on-call pay, and other factors that may affect department salary expense.

Exhibit 6–3 Community Hospital Personnel Requirements Worksheet

---

19X0 Budget Request

Department: _____

Position: _____

Biweekly Hours: _____   Date Needed: _____

What created this need?

What will happen if the requested change is not approved?

Fringe Benefits

Mandated benefits as a percentage of salary expense normally increase slightly each year because of scheduled increases in Social Security, workmen's compensation, or unemployment compensation. Hospital-controlled fringe benefits—such as hospitalization, life insurance, retirement, and paid days off (holidays, vacations, sick-leave days)—do not change as a percentage of salary unless the hospital makes a significant change in its policy. Therefore, if salary expense increases ten percent, mandated benefits will increase slightly more than ten percent, and hospital controlled benefits will increase approximately ten percent.

Most hospitals budget fringe benefits as a percentage of salary expense. Although many hospitals budget fringe benefits in a lump sum, there is a growing trend toward budgeting, as well as recording, fringe benefits by department. Department analysis is improved when fringe benefits are departmentalized because there is a better matching of revenues with expenses by period.

Fringe benefits as a percentage of salary should be one of the hospital's assumptions.

Budget Hearings

After the department heads have prepared their proposed changes in the position control and their nonsalary requests, the controller should schedule budget hearings. As previously noted in the section on the budget calendar, those present should include the controller, the administrator or assistant administrator, and the department head.

At a budget hearing, the first task is to get all parties to agree that the request is reasonable. The controller should have Monitrend statistics, comparisons with other area hospitals, and any other comparable data that have been collected. The budget request should be negotiated between the department heads and their administrative superior with the controller acting only as a facilitator. The most difficult task of the controller will be to keep the hearing on a rational basis. The department heads will have a tendency to justify the status quo because they have a vested interest in present operations. If the administrator does not have a strong accounting background, there will be a tendency to use intuition or to rely excessively on past experience. As a facilitator, the controller will refer to documented examples, statistical data, and the parameters established by the budget assumptions.

During the budget hearing, it is important to keep in mind that hospitals have three major categories of expenses. These are committed fixed costs, discretionary fixed costs, and variable costs.

Committed fixed costs are costs that would continue even if the hospital were closed. In a bankruptcy proceeding, committed fixed costs would be included in the creditors' claims. Some examples of committed fixed costs are payments on long-term debt, certain lease payments, and amounts due under a noncancelable contract.

Discretionary fixed costs are costs that the hospital has selected to become fixed costs. Since the hospital has chosen to identify these costs as fixed costs, the hospital can decide to make them variable, to eliminate them, or to reduce them. Some examples of discretionary fixed costs are all salaried payroll expense, a great deal of hourly payroll expense, costs of 24-hour coverage for emergency room and delivery room, all lease agreements that are not committed fixed costs, amounts due under a cancelable contract, all service and maintenance agreements, insurance, nongovernmental-mandated fringe benefits, most printing and photocopy costs, and physician contracts. Most hospital operating expenses can be classified as discretionary fixed costs. Most hospital costs that can be reduced, either with or without a corresponding reduction in patient care, are expenses that the hospital has chosen to make fixed for the budget period.

Variable costs are costs that increase or decrease with the volume of patients treated. Some examples of variable costs are all hourly payroll expense that is not discretionary fixed cost, supply and drug costs, utilities, some fringe benefits, some malpractice insurance, chemicals, contracts that are based on volume of service, and other costs that vary with changes in the number of patients treated. Reductions can be made in variable costs only by reducing either the quality of patient care or patient comfort and convenience. Often the quality of care for a particular patient service is too high, or patient comfort and convenience is at a level that is not reasonable. In these instances, the hospital should reduce the applicable unit variable costs.

The controller should not make decisions regarding discretionary fixed costs or the level of patient care outside of the controller's area. However, the controller can and should influence these decisions by making sure that administration as well as department heads clearly understand the differences between committed fixed costs, discretionary fixed costs, and variable costs. It is also the responsibility of the chief financial officer to explain the expense options available through the budget process.

Throughout the budget hearings, it is important for administration, the controller, and the hospital board member, if one is present, to keep in mind that the budget assumptions are based on facts known at the time the budget is being prepared. During the budget period, certain events or circumstances will occur that could not have been anticipated in advance. Because of third party payer constraints—such as reimbursement under the lower of costs or charges and the constraints of external rate-setting processes—the hospital must guard its financial viability through deliberate overbudgeting in some expense categories. Deliberate overbudgeting must always be in expense categories that either will not be abused by department managers or that are completely controlled by administration. The following are areas in which deliberate overbudgeting can be effective: bad debt expense, contractual allowances, fringe benefits, departments where it is known that the manager will not spend more than necessary in spite of favorable budget variances, categories such as travel expense if administration can control such expense through an administrative policy (i.e., prior approval required before all hospital-reimbursed travel), utilities, insurance, and other expense areas that are not directly controlled by department heads.

At least 30 minutes should be scheduled for each budget hearing. If the first draft of the department request is tentatively approved in less than 30 minutes, the time can be used to dictate or write a summary of the budget hearing.

The Master Budget

After the budget hearings are completed, the tentatively approved departmental requests must be summarized into the master expense budget for the hospital. The master expense budget is summarized by program or by major expense category for the entire hospital and compared to the current year's projected expense or to the current year's budget. Each line of this comparison should be examined for reasonableness.

This first draft of the consolidated expense budget should be presented to the administrator or to the budget committee with an estimate of the average price increase necessary to fund the budget and at the same time achieve the targeted net gain. If the average price increase appears reasonable as well as achievable, the controller can begin the revenue budget. If the needed price increase is not reasonable, the controller must propose areas, functions, or categories of budgeted expenses that can be cut. Although the expenses proposed to be cut will depend upon the individual hospital and on the prevailing circumstances, it should be noted that at this point in the budget process most reductions will be made either in discretionary costs or in those categories of expense that are deliberately overbudgeted.

Other Budget Items

In addition to the departmental budgets, the hospital will have several items that affect the entire hospital. These include, but are not limited to, depreciation, planned consulting fees, pension plan benefits, interest expense, and other expenses of an administrative nature. These are normally budgeted by the controller.

If the hospital is partially or totally committed to a variable budget, the budget process must examine costs per unit of service for both salary expense and nonsalary expense. With variable budgeting, the department head makes two separate adjustments to historical data. The first is for workload, which may be an increase or a decrease in the base data. The second is for inflation. With variable budgeting, the budgeted increase for inflation is segregated from changes for volume in order to provide a means of separating the two in analyzing budget variances. All variances are broken into their volume component and their price component.

COMPREHENSIVE BUDGET PHILOSOPHIES

In the past several years, many comprehensive budget philosophies have been lauded. This section briefly examines three of these comprehensive philosophies. They are management by objectives, zero-based budgeting, and program budgeting.

Management by Objectives

Management by objectives presupposes a structured organization chart with well-defined policies, procedures, goals, and objectives. The best way to explain how management by objectives works in a hospital setting is to walk through an implementation example. The following example assumes that the hospital has a functioning participatory budget system. If the department heads have not participated in budget preparation and in variance analysis for their departments, the hospital will need to spend one or two years developing these skills in the department managers.

The first task in preparing for management by objectives is to have each department develop a departmental charter. This charter defines the reason for that department's existence and shows how this blends into the mission of the hospital. If the hospital board has defined a corporate mission, the department charter can make reference to this. If the hospital does not have an approved corporate mission, the manager writing the department charter will have to make certain assumptions regarding the hospital's mission. The department charters must be reviewed and approved by the administrator or some other hospital official. In developing the charter for each department, a person knowledgeable in management-by-objectives techniques should be available for assistance. This person will actually have to write the first draft of many of the charters.

Once the departmental charters are completed, the department heads will be familiar with concepts such as mission and departmental goals versus institutional goals. They will also have had the opportunity of negotiating their department charter. With this orientation, they can benefit from formal instruction in management-by-objectives principles and techniques. All department heads should be required to attend such hospital-sponsored instruction. This should be tailormade for the particular hospital and be given by a consultant, professional educator, or other person who has established teaching skills and management-by-objectives experience. Management by objectives has failed in many hospitals because either department heads or administration did not understand the basic principles. It is very difficult to initiate this budget philosophy without formal education for both department managers and administration.

As department heads prepare their budget requests, they also prepare a draft of several objectives that they hope to accomplish during the budget period. These objectives must be descriptive enough to be measurable or they cannot be negotiated. To say the hospital will reduce infections is not a measurable objective. This can be reworded to state that there will be 40 percent fewer positive cultures from routine infection control samples and that this will be accomplished by midyear. To state that patient billing will improve is not measurable and, therefore, not an acceptable goal. This can be reworded to state that the average billing lag from date of discharge to date of billing will be reduced by one day by the end of the first quarter and by an additional two days by the end of the second quarter. An objective from a department is not sufficiently defined to negotiate until it is measurable. It would be helpful to supply copies of management-by-objectives forms with instructions. A sample worksheet is shown in Exhibit 6–4.

In the worksheet, the objective is what the department proposes to accomplish, and a critical issue is an event that must happen or a decision that must be made before the objective can be met. Not all objectives have a critical issue.

It is important for the supervisor to remember that activities are not objectives. Objectives are output-oriented and serve as a performance measurement for the department. An objective identifies something the department will accomplish

Exhibit 6–4 Community Hospital Management-by-Objectives Worksheet

		Date	
		Begin	Complete
Objective	Critical Issue		

For the Year Ended December 31, 19XX

to improve its performance; establishes a specific time, such as the month or quarter, by which the department plans to accomplish this; and is capable of being measured.

The proposed objectives must be negotiated under the managers' supervision. In this negotiation process, money and other resources needed to support the objectives are discussed. If an objective is not affordable, it is either rejected or postponed until another budget period. In the negotiation process, the reasonableness of each proposed objective must also be discussed. Some proposed objectives will be too easy, and the supervisor will have to negotiate objectives that are not so easily attainable. Other proposed objectives will be unattainable, and the supervisor will need to reduce them down to a more realistic level.

Once administration and the department head have agreed on a set of objectives, the objectives become something like a management contract. The department's commitment is to achieve the agreed-upon goals and objectives. Administration's commitment is to blend these objectives into the goals and objectives of the hospital, to provide the resources needed to meet the objectives, and to support them in every possible way.

After management by objectives is functioning between administration and department heads, the hospital should initiate this tool between department heads and first-line supervisors as well as between first-line supervisors and employees. Experience has shown that management by objectives works best when achievement of the negotiated goals directly affects the employees' annual merit pay increases.

It must be emphasized that management by objectives is a style of management that allows goals and objectives to be proposed and negotiated at as low an administrative level as possible. It cannot work unless the administrator and assistant administrator are fully committed to allowing decisions to be made at the department level. Management by objectives has failed in many hospitals because top management was unable to allow decisions to be made at the lower level. Before initiating management by objectives, the hospital's senior administrators should carefully assess their willingness to relinquish enough control over department goal-setting to make the system work. If the answer is no or maybe, then some other budget philosophy should be chosen for their hospital.

Zero-Based Budgeting

Zero-based budgeting in hospitals can best be described as an approach to planning and budgeting. The word *approach* is important because zero-based budgeting cannot be applied as a hard and fast technique in hospitals. In this section we will examine the basic concepts of this approach in the hospital setting.

The first task needed to implement zero-based budgeting is to define goals and objectives first for the hospital, then for identifiable functions, such as nursing services; ancillary services; general support; administrative support; and providing, maintaining, and cleaning plant facilities. The objectives for the identifiable major functions will define the service level for each of these activities. A service level is a broad qualitative objective; for example:

- bills for inpatient service will be mailed no later than nine days after discharge

- central supply lost-charge slips will equal about two percent of gross revenue for a particular department

- the pharmacy will dispense medication with a unit-dose system and will have an admixture program for intervenous solutions

- the laboratory will do 90 percent of the diagnostic tests in-house and refer 10 percent to an outside laboratory.

Once goals and objectives have been defined for the major functions necessary to operate the hospital, a list of activities and subactivities for each of the major functions must be developed to show exactly what is needed to perform the functions at the desired service level. This list of activities and the defined service levels must be developed with input from the department heads.

Once the goals, activities, subactivities, and service levels for each department have been identified, the department managers are expected to tell what resources and personnel are needed to achieve them. The hospital must take the position that the number of people the department had in similar activities in the past is unequivocally irrelevant. It is critical that managers do not look at existing resources and staffing and say, okay, we need that much plus ten percent. Incremental budgeting must be rejected from the outset. At this point, departments know what they are expected to do and need only define what is needed to accomplish it.

The basic budget document used in zero-based budgeting is called a decision package. The department head prepares a decision package for each current or proposed function or activity that has been defined. The decision package identifies the resources and personnel needed to perform that activity at the minimum level needed, the current level if this is an existing function, and other appropriate levels. In the decision package these levels are related to expected benefits.

Once the department budget requests are broken down into decision packages, the department manager gives each decision unit a priority ranking and submits the budget proposal to administration. Administration has a unique vantage point and brings this broader perspective to bear in making program tradeoffs. At this higher level, priority ranking is changed and programs can be added, deleted, or revised.

Hospitals do not put money into savings accounts. Funds are either spent for needed services or the hospital reduces its planned rate increase. Because of this, hospitals have a great need for goal congruence. Zero-based budgeting gives the board, as well as administration, a unique opportunity to get involved in building the operating budgets rather than just reviewing them.

Although this budget approach can provide a degree of integration between operating plans and financial plans that is seldom achieved in most hospitals, it will not work and should not be tried in every institution. It is an approach that requires a commitment from the chief executive officer. This executive must be not only interested in zero-based budgeting but must be personally supportive. This budget approach takes a lot of effort and is very difficult and time-consuming to implement.

It should also be cautioned that the accomplishments of zero-based budgeting are difficult to measure in specific monetary terms. Much of the benefit takes place at the level of the decision packages as department heads evaluate and redirect their resources to achieve better goal congruence.

Program Budgeting

Program budgeting is a unique technique for evaluating the hospital's budget as well as analyzing variances. Although program budgeting is most often associated with an incremental approach to departmental budgeting, with some modifications it can also be used effectively in conjunction with zero-based budgeting, management by objectives, and other budget philosophies.

To initiate program budgeting, the hospital must first define its programs or major classifications of revenue and expense. A list of budget or decision programs for a hospital could include inpatient care, outpatient care, ancillary services, general services, plant services, administrative, and general. Within each of these programs the hospital could have subprograms.

As the department heads submit their line-item budgets, their requests are summarized by program. The budgets are not evaluated in terms of salary expense, supply expense, utilities, travel, and other expense classifications. Instead, the budget is evaluated in terms of inpatient care, ancillary services, plant services, and other programs. Rather than trying to determine how much supply costs to budget, the hospital makes decisions on questions like, how much should we spend on outpatient services next year? Program budgeting thus is merely a traditional budget preparation exercise, but the end result is evaluated differently. At the departmental level, there is little or no difference.

Although program budgeting can be used by any hospital, it works best in an institution that has carefully defined annual goals and objectives. If these goals and objectives have been identified for several years into the future, the administrator can identify programs by the year in which the hospital will place a major budget emphasis. By evaluating the hospital's present strengths and weaknesses by year, a plan can be formulated to correct these over time. Program budgeting is a superior way to manage goal congruence because it is geared to top management thinking.

Just as other budget philosophies should be implemented only if they conform to the thinking and management style of the chief executive officer, program budgeting should not be used unless the administrator is willing to make decisions by program.

SUMMARY

The hospital budget process is not unlike the budget process of an individual, a small business, or a large chain of businesses. In each of these processes we make choices because of limited funds. As the organization becomes more complex, it requires a more formal budget process. As the organization becomes larger, more people are required to produce an effective budget. All hospitals today are complex entities as well as big business enterprises. No hospital can have a workable budget without departmental input.

The budget process begins with a budget calendar that becomes the roadmap through the entire process. The process then generates budget assumptions that set the parameters and define the goals for the budget period. The department heads are given historical information and whatever assistance they need to prepare budget requests. Budget hearings are held and typed summaries are made of the hearings.

Throughout the budget process, it should be kept in mind that hospitals have three kinds of costs to consider in the annual operating budget. The first is variable costs, which vary directly with workload. Hospitals also have two kinds of fixed costs. There are committed fixed costs over which the hospital no longer has any control. Control of committed fixed costs is exercised only when the costs are incurred. The other type of fixed cost is discretionary fixed cost. Discretionary fixed costs are costs that the hospital has chosen to make fixed. In budgeting and planning, cost control is exercised by making discretionary fixed all costs that could be either committed fixed or discretionary fixed. Costs that can be either discretionary fixed or variable should be made variable.

Many hospitals have adopted comprehensive budget philosophies. To be effective, these philosophies must support the management style and operating philosophy of the hospital's administration. In this chapter we have examined management by objectives, zero-based budgeting, and program budgeting.

DISCUSSION QUESTIONS

1. Discuss some of the reasons why the administrator and the controller should not prepare the hospital budget without departmental input.
2. List the major steps in a good hospital budget process.
3. How should department heads prepare for a budget hearing? How should the controller prepare?
4. Explain how deliberate overbudgeting in some expense categories can be used as an effective management tool.
5. How is a position control used to budget and to control salaries and wages?
6. What is the difference between committed fixed costs and discretionary fixed costs?
7. Briefly define management by objectives, zero-based budgeting, and program budgeting.

Chapter 7

Budgeting Revenue and Pricing Strategy

In Chapter 6 we discussed expense budgeting. In this chapter we will complete the analysis of the current year's operating budget by examining revenue budgets and pricing strategy.

Statistical Budgets

We have already touched upon the statistical budget in our discussion of budget assumptions. Before examining revenue budgets, we will look at statistical budgeting more closely. Statistical budgets are the foundation upon which all revenue budgets are built.

Patient Days

The most important statistic for hospitals is patient days. Other statistics are either directly tied to or are subordinate to patient days. Patient days should be forecast first in total, then by month, and finally monthly by nursing station. The methodology enumerated in this section can be used as a guide.

The first step is to develop historical patient-day statistics by type of service. The hospital should show at least two years of actual data and a projection of the current year's patient days. Table 7–1 is an example of a form used to formalize the projection.

In addition to historical data, the hospital must consider other factors that affect patient days. These include expected changes in number of staff physicians, population trends in the hospital's primary service area, age of population in the primary service area, economic projections in the hospital's primary service area, projected changes in third party coverage such as increased benefits under Medicare or Medicaid, and other factors. Depending upon the size of the hospital and the complexity of the many factors that affect patient days, con-

Table 7-1 Community Hospital Comparative Patient-Days Statistics

Budget Year 19X1
Year Ended Dec. 31

Service	Actual 19W8	Actual 19W9	Projected 19X0	Forecast 19X1
Nursery	XX	XX	XX	
Obstetrics	XX	XX	XX	
Pediatrics	XX	XX	XX	
Medical	XX	XX	XX	
Surgical	XX	XX	XX	
Coronary	XX	XX	XX	
Intensive	XX	XX	XX	
Total	XXX	XXX	XXX	

sideration of these assumptions can range from an informal discussion with the medical staff to a well-defined documented process.

After total patient days by service have been forecast, the hospital must convert the annual forecast into a monthly forecast. One of the most effective ways to accomplish this is to study historical patient days by month. If more than two years are compared, a weighted average should be used to minimize the error of using trends that are no longer relevant. In addition to historical trends, the hospital should consider any other factors that may have an effect on the monthly usage of hospital days by each service.

The monthly patient-days budget by service should be projected by nursing unit and a forecasted percent occupancy by unit calculated. The projection by nursing unit is used to establish personnel requirements, to schedule vacations and other paid days off, and to determine which nursing units, if any, should be closed during projected periods of low census.

Outpatient Occasions of Service

There are four major types of outpatient occasions of service to consider. These are emergency room visits that become inpatients, emergency room visits that are ambulatory, referred outpatients, and clinics. Because emergency room visits that result in an admission are significantly and measurably more acute than emergency room visits that are ambulatory, it is useful to project these outpatient occasions of service separately. Referred outpatients are patients who come to the hospital to receive a specific test or treatment prescribed by their physicians. Although the most commonly referred outpatients are in radiology and the laboratory, many other departments—such as electroencephalography, electrocardiology, physical therapy, and speech pathology—perform services for patients referred by staff or other community doctors. Clinic visits are not available at all hospitals. However, if the hospital does provide general and/or specialized clinic services, these must be forecast as a distinct category of outpatient occasion of service.

To project outpatient occasions of service by class of service, the hospital must first project historical data by class of service. The historical data are used in conjunction with known or expected changes in the medical staff, mix of patients, physical facilities, medical or technological advancements, other outpatient facilities, population growth, and other factors to project occasions of service for the budget period. This is then converted to a monthly forecast by class of service.

Ancillary Services

Patient days and outpatient occasions of service form the foundation from which ancillary service statistics are forecast. In this section we will examine two methods of forecasting these statistics. The methodology used by the individual hospital will depend on the training and background of the department heads as well as the particular needs of the hospital.

The first method of estimating ancillary department revenue is to present the historical and projected patient days and outpatient occasions of service statistics to the department heads and ask them to estimate a percentage increase or decrease in revenue for their departments at current year prices. It is important that the projections be at current year prices since pricing strategy will not be developed until later in the budget process.

The estimated percentage change is applied to the current year's projected revenue to estimate gross revenue in the budget period at current prices. This method is straightforward and easily understood by department heads.

If the hospital needs a more precise forecast for rate-setting review, for presentation to a committee of the board, or for management, historical data by patient day and by outpatient occasion of service should be prepared for each ancillary service. Table 7–2 is an example of a statistical forecast worksheet for the laboratory. A similar worksheet should be prepared for each ancillary.

Using the statistical worksheet in conjunction with their knowledge of departmental trends, department managers can forecast tests or procedures per inpatient day and per outpatient occasion of service by month. It is important to forecast these statistics by month in order to project any predictable seasonal trends in ancillary department statistics.

Table 7-2 Community Hospital Statistical Forecast Worksheet

Laboratory—Budget Year 19X1

	Tests Per Patient Day			Tests Per OP Occasion		
	Actual 19W9	Actual 19X0	Forecast 19X1	Actual 19W9	Actual 19X0	Forecast 19X1
January	XX	XX		XX	XX	
February	XX	XX		XX	XX	
March	XX	XX		XX	XX	
↓	↓	↓		↓	↓	
December	XX	XX		XX	XX	
Total	XXX	XXX		XXX	XXX	

After tests or procedures per unit of service have been forecast for each ancillary, the statistics are multiplied by the applicable inpatient days and out-patient occasions of service by month. This method takes considerably more time than estimating percentage change in revenue at constant prices as described earlier. However, the forecast is generally more accurate, and budget variances can be explained more understandably.

REVENUE BUDGETS

Because of the nature of hospital services, the statistical budget and the expense budget must be completed before the revenue budgets can be started. This is particularly important in the case of cost-based reimbursement. In the first section of this chapter we studied statistical budgets; expense budgets were covered in Chapter 6. In this section we will examine revenue budgets.

Foundation for Revenue Budgets

Budgeting revenue in hospitals is the mechanical process of taking the rate structure on targeted gain, adding expected expenses to arrive at targeted net revenue, adding allowances and adjustments to determine targeted gross revenue, and finally raising prices to reach the targeted gross revenue. This is expressed in the following formula:

$$BR = EG + FE + AA$$

where:

$$BR = \text{budgeted revenue}$$
$$EG = \text{expected gain}$$
$$FE = \text{forecasted expenses}$$
$$AA = \text{allowances and adjustments}$$

We will examine separately each of the three components that make up budgeted revenue.

Expected gain is the amount of gain the hospital needs to fulfill working capital requirements, prepare for eventual replacement of equipment and physical plant, keep up with appropriate technology, and provide for sound financial operations. Numerous hospitals fail to budget enough gain. The board or the administrator of these hospitals believe that profit is a dirty word and feel a community obligation to budget as close to breakeven as possible. However, a hospital that operates at breakeven for a number of years is either heading toward financial disaster or is borrowing from the future. Medical technology advances every year, and if the hospital does not systematically chase new technology it will lose the loyalty of its medical staff. In addition, the hospital must replace existing technology at inflated prices.

The amount of net gain to be budgeted each year should include such subjective considerations as long-range pricing strategy, national as well as local economic forecasts, long-range capital budgets, and known or expected legislation or regulations that will effect the hospital. The hospital must also budget enough net gain to offset any adverse changes in cost-based reimbursement formulas and utilization.

The second component in the formula for budgeting revenue, forecasted expenses, was covered in the previous chapter. Here it should be added that, in budgeting revenue, the hospital adjusts the expense budget for any deliberate overbudgeting in order to get a true picture of expected net gain. If the hospital does not undergo a comprehensive budget-and-rate review process with an outside agency, the amount of hidden deliberate overbudgeting will be just enough to cover contingencies. If the hospital must go through a very comprehensive rate review process, the amount of deliberate overbudgeting will include a buffer to protect its financial base. Depending upon the motives for and the amount of deliberate overbudgeting, the hospital may adjust budgeted expenses significantly, or it may make no adjustment to budgeted expenses in the rate-setting process.

The third component of the budgeted revenue formula is allowances and adjustments. This includes forecasted bad debts, free care, charity, contractual adjustments for cost reports, other contractual adjustments, discounts, and other revenue deductions. The most difficult revenue deductions to predict are cost-based, third party payer contractual deductions. The concept of these contractual adjustments is explained fully in the chapter on reimbursement.

After the hospital has defined and understands expected gain, forecasted expenses, and allowances and adjustments for the budget period, it has the foundation for a sound revenue budget. The overall pricing strategy can now be determined.

Average Price Increase

The overall pricing strategy is comprised of three components. These are average price increase, departmental price increase, and individual-procedure price increase.

Before calculating the overall average price increase, the expected budget period's patient gross revenue at current year's prices must be known. This is done departmentally by multiplying the work-level assumptions developed in the statistical budget by the current year's prices. The projected gross revenue by department is then totaled to obtain total patient revenue at current year's prices. By studying a simple proforma profit and loss statement for the budget period, we can calculate the projected overall hospital price increase. The proforma statement for Community Hospital in Table 7–3 can be used as a guide.

At this point, we know the targeted net gain and the budgeted expenses. Adding these together gives total net income. Other income is now subtracted from total net income to obtain net patient revenue. Allowances and adjustments are then added to net patient revenue to obtain gross patient revenue. From this, patient revenue at current year's prices is subtracted to obtain gross revenue from price increases. This can be expressed in the following formula:

$$PI = NG + BE + AA - OI - CP$$

where:

        PI = Patient revenue from price increases
        NG = Net gain (loss)
        BE = Budgeted expenses
        AA = Allowances and adjustments
        OI = Other income
        CP = Patient revenue at current year's prices

The patient revenue from price increases should be expressed as a percent of patient revenue at current year's prices. The patient revenue at current year's prices includes an adjustment for changes in workloads. The percentage derived, therefore, includes only the projected average overall price increase. This percentage must be examined for reasonableness. If the needed percentage increase is not attainable because of mandated or negotiable constraints of outside agen-

Table 7–3 Community Hospital Proforma Statement of Profit and Loss

Budget Period Ended Dec. 31, 19X0

Patient revenue:	
At current year's prices	$XXXX
From price increases	XX
Total gross patient revenue	XXXX
Less allowances and adjustments	XX
Net Patient Revenue	XXXX
Other income	XX
Total net income	XXXX
Less expenses	XXXX
Net gain (loss)	$ XX

cies, board or administrative philosophy, economic climate, or other impediment, then the hospital must decrease either net gain or budgeted expenses. It must be cautioned that these changes will not have a dollar-for-dollar effect on revenue because of cost-based reimbursement. It is necessary to recalculate contractual allowances each time a change is made in net gain or budgeted expenses and to rework the formula to determine a new average percent price increase.

Departmental Price Increases

There are many computer programs available to maximize net revenue once the hospital has budgeted an overall net gain. All of the large certified public accounting firms either have a computer simulation model to assist their clients with pricing strategy or have access to a simulation model on a timesharing basis. In addition, many consultants, shared-service data-processing firms, and hospital associations have access to a computer model to assist in pricing strategy. This section will illustrate some general principles governing the use of these models and will provide enough understanding of pricing to enable hospitals that do not have access to a simulation model to develop a pricing strategy.

The first requirement in determining departmental price increases is to allocate nonrevenue producing departments to revenue producing departments. This allocation is intended to approximate the step-down allocation used for third-party payer cost reports. This allocation can be estimated by developing ratios to the budgeted expenses for all revenue departments. More accurate information can be obtained by completing an actual step-down using budgeted information. This step-down can be completed in less than one day. The additional usefulness and accuracy of the information normally justify completing a step-down and doing a set of minicost reports on budgeted data.

The allocation process determines the total amount of cost that a revenue department must cover just to break even. The next step is to establish a cost-reimbursed departmental ranking schedule using the most current revenue-by-payer information that is available for a period long enough to compensate for seasonal fluctuations. This is usually the last fiscal year.

To establish a department ranking schedule, the controller determines the percent of revenue for each department that is cost reimbursed. Cost-reimbursed revenue includes Medicare, Medicaid, in many states Blue Cross, and other programs. The departments are then ranked with the lowest percentage cost-reimbursed department first and the highest percentage cost-reimbursed department last. An example of a department ranking schedule for Community Hospital is shown in Table 7–4.

In the Table 7–4 example, for every $1.00 of gross revenue that the hospital generates through price increases in private room rates, it can collect a maximum of $.68 and will book at least $.32 in contractual adjustments. For every $1.00 of gross revenue generated through price increases in the coronary care room rate, the hospital can only collect a maximum of $.46 and will book at least $.54 in contractual adjustments. Cost-based payers are not affected by hospital price increases because the amount they pay is based on a cost report, not billed charges. The hospital can increase net revenue only by raising prices to patients who pay billed charges.

With a stepdown and a departmental ranking completed, the hospital is ready to make the first draft of a departmental price increase schedule. This first draft

Table 7–4 Community Hospital Department Ranking Schedule

| | | Percent of Revenue Which Is | |
| | | Charge | Cost |
Revenue Center	Rank	Reimbursed	Reimbursed
Private room	1	68%	32%
⋮			
Nuclear medicine	28	65%	35%
Physical therapy	29	64%	36%
Laboratory	30	60%	40%
Intensive care	31	57%	43%
Semiprivate	32	55%	45%
EKG	33	53%	47%
Radiology	34	51%	49%
Coronary care	35	46%	54%

Table 7-5 Community Hospital Departmental Price Increase Worksheet

1	2	3	4	5	6	7	8	9	10	11
Rank	Department	Direct Cost	+ Allocated Cost =	Total Cost	+ Markup On Cost =	Needed Net Revenue	+ Add Allowances Adjustments =	Needed Gross Revenue	Revenue With No Price Increase	Average Percent Price Increase
1	Private room	$ XX	$ XX	$ XXX	$ X	$ XXX	$ XX	$ XXX	$ XXX	10%
28	Nuclear medicine	XX	XX	XXX	X	XXX	XX	XXX	XXX	8
29	Physical therapy	XX	XX	XXX	X	XXX	XX	XXX	XXX	8
30	Laboratory	XX	XX	XXX	X	XXX	XX	XXX	XXX	5
31	Intensive care	XX	XX	XXX	X	XXX	XX	XXX	XXX	11
32	Semiprivate	XX	XX	XXX	X	XXX	XX	XXX	XXX	14
33	EKG	XX	XX	XXX	X	XXX	XX	XXX	XXX	8
34	Radiology	XX	XX	XXX	X	XXX	XX	XXX	XXX	6
35	Coronary care	XX	XX	XXX	X	XXX	XX	XXX	XXX	10
	Total all departments	XXXX	XXXX	XXXXX	XXX	XXXXX	XXXX	XXXXX	XXXXX	8%

should assume that every department will have the same percentage markup on total costs. Table 7–5 is an example of a departmental price increase worksheet for Community Hospital. This example is purposefully detailed in order to illustrate the theory and logic of assigning departmental price increases.

The revenue-producing departments are listed on the departmental price increase worksheet in the order they appear on the ranking schedule illustrated in Table 7–4. This makes us mindful of the fact that the hospital will gain the most net revenue by assigning the highest markup on cost to those departments that have the greatest percentage of charge-reimbursed revenue. Column three on the Table 7–5 worksheet represents budgeted direct cost for each department. Allocated cost represents the cost of the nonrevenue producing departments that have been allocated in the step-down process. Total cost in column five represents the total of columns three and four.

Markup on cost in column six should represent the same percentage markup for each department. This percentage is calculated by taking the budgeted net gain from Table 7–3 and dividing this by the total budgeted cost for the hospital from column five. Needed net revenue by department is the sum of total cost plus markup on cost. If all revenue departments cover their proportionate share of nonrevenue departmental overhead, allowances and adjustments are added to net revenue to obtain needed gross revenue by department.

By dividing departmental needed gross revenue in column nine by what revenue is projected to be if the hospital implemented no price increase, the average percentage price increase needed by department is revealed. In our hypothetical example, the room-and-board rates require a larger increase than the ancillary departments. Laboratory and radiology in our example require a smaller increase than the other ancillaries. This implies that room-and-board rates in the past have been kept relatively low and that this has been compensated for by pricing the laboratory and radiology high.

Having calculated the required average price increase by department to equalize net gain among all of the revenue producing departments, the hospital is prepared to begin departmental pricing strategy. Without changing the overall average price increase or the budgeted net gain, tradeoffs can be made between departments. Our hypothetical example in Table 7–5 indicated the hospital should consider raising its semiprivate room rate by 14 percent, the intensive care room rate by 11 percent, and the coronary care and private room rate by 10 percent. It would be very unusual for a hospital to raise its semiprivate room rate 14 percent in one year. It would also be unusual for a hospital to raise its other room rates by the amounts indicated. Even if public pressures and prevailing rates at other area hospitals and other factors that caused the hospital to keep room rates relatively low in the past have changed, past pricing policies cannot be changed in a single year.

At this point, the hospital's chief financial officer and chief executive officer should meet to determine departmental price tradeoffs. Should the ancillary departments be priced high in order to keep room rates relatively low? How much higher, if any, should the departments with a high percentage of billed-charges revenue be priced? What pricing strategy should the hospital follow over five years, and how can current pricing lead into this five-year plan? How can pricing be used to maximize net revenue in view of current as well as proposed regulations and controls? These and other questions must be either formally or intuitively addressed by the hospital's administration.

Tradeoffs between departments must be made in dollar amounts and then converted to average percent price increases. In our example, assume the decision is made to increase semiprivate room rates by only nine percent and to increase laboratory revenue enough to offset the resulting loss. Assume further that the selected amounts from our worksheet in Table 7–5 are as follows:

Department	*Needed Gross Revenue*	*Revenue With No Price Increase*	*Average Percent Price Increase*
Laboratory	$1,050,000	$1,000,000	5
Semiprivate	3,990,000	3,500,000	14

A 9.0 percent increase in the semiprivate room rate would generate $3,815,000 in gross revenue, which is $175,000 less than gross revenue with a 14.0 percent increase. Adding $175,000 to the needed gross revenue in laboratory gives us $1,225,000 needed gross revenue. To achieve the required new gross revenue, the average percent price increase in the laboratory would be 22.5 percent. Revised selected amounts from our Table 7–5 worksheet are as follows:

Department	*Needed Gross Revenue*	*Revenue With No Price Increase*	*Average Percent Price Increase*
Laboratory	$1,225,000	$1,000,000	22.5
Semiprivate	3,815,000	3,500,000	9.0

The hospital must now determine whether the 22.5 percent increase in laboratory prices is attainable. This increase is probably not attainable for any one of several reasons. The physicians won't accept it, third party payers won't accept it, or the hospital board or the public won't accept it. The chief executive and the chief financial officer must then take part of the increase away from the laboratory and give it to another department. This process continues until the average price increase for each department is attainable as well as acceptable.

It is important throughout the departmental pricing strategy to be mindful of the department charge-reimbursed ranking. Whenever possible, the high-ranking departments should have a higher markup on total cost than the low-ranking departments. This does not mean that high-ranking departments will receive the highest percentage increase. If pricing strategy in prior years has been effective, the hospital already will be maximizing net revenue through departmental mark-ups, and the average percentage price increase will be approximately equal for each department.

Individual Procedure Price Increase

In the previous section, the average departmental price increase was determined. In this section, we shall examine how to determine which tests, procedures, or items within each department should have a larger-than-average markup. The purpose of pricing strategy within each department is to maximize net income.

Before initiating pricing strategy to maximize income, the individual department heads should be asked to identify any test or procedure that is priced either excessively high or excessively low. Often the hospital will have a procedure that is currently priced significantly differently than the identical test performed in other area or regional hospitals. Sometimes a department head will feel that a particular test is priced so low that the hospital is losing money. For every test or procedure reported by a department to be significantly mispriced, the accounting department should calculate a price as if the charge item were a new test. In the next section, we will show how to determine the price for a new test or service.

If it is found that the charge item is significantly overpriced, the price should be frozen for one or more years. If it is found that the charge item is significantly underpriced, the price should be increased enough to compensate. The hospital should now go back to the departmental price-ranking schedule. For those departments that are more than 50 percent cost reimbursed, the hospital will maximize net income by pricing higher those tests or procedures that are performed predominately on cost-reimbursed patients than the tests performed predominately on charge-reimbursed patients. To illustrate this concept, assume a department that is presently 70-percent cost reimbursed, has direct plus indirect expenses of $200,000 on the cost report, and has $250,000 of gross patient revenue. Assume further that there is a test that is almost always performed on a Medicare patient and is, therefore, 100 percent cost reimbursed. If the revenue from this test is presently $20,000, reimbursement for this department can be increased as follows:

Present reimbursement:

$$\frac{.70 \times 200,000}{200,000} \times 250,000 = \$175,000$$

If price of this test increased by \$5,000:

$$\frac{(.70 \times 200,000) + (1.00 \times 5,000)}{205,000} \times 250,000 = \$176,800$$

In this example, because the department is highly cost reimbursed and we chose a test that is totally Medicare reimbursed, the hospital will receive \$1,768 more in "cost reimbursement."

Most cost reports utilize the ratio of program charges to total charges against cost, or RCCAC. The hospital in our example can maximize allowable cost by adopting a pricing strategy that makes the RCCAC as large as practical.

This section can be summarized by citing two rules of thumb. If the department is highly cost reimbursed, the prices of cost-reimbursed tests should be kept relatively high. If the department is highly billed-charges reimbursed, the prices of billed charges tests should be kept relatively high. If the hospital has access to a computer simulation model to use in its pricing, the amount of gain from this strategy can be estimated. If the hospital does not have access to a simulation model, the pricing must be done intuitively. It should be cautioned that gains made from pricing strategy will be relatively small when expressed as a percentage of total net revenue. Large gains either would not be approved in the hospital's rate review or would indicate that the hospital has arbitrarily set prices in a fraudulent manner. This does not mean that some hospitals should ignore pricing strategy. A one percent gain in net revenue for a hospital that has ten million dollars in net revenue is one hundred thousand dollars.

Price by Formula

In many regions, a hospital's prices for pharmacy and central supply are based on a formula rather than a stated amount for each item. For example, the price might be:

Hospital Cost	*Patient Cost*
\$0 – \$10.00	Cost times 200%
\$10.01 – \$50.00	Cost times 175%
\$50.01 – \$200.00	Cost times 150%
Over \$200.00	Cost plus \$100.00

If the formula is mandated by a rate-review committee, by a major third party payer, or by the Medicare intermediary, the only action the hospital can take to maximize reimbursement is to increase prices to patients as soon as the hospital's supplier increases the cost to the hospital. A delay in increasing prices results in a potential revenue loss equal to not only the increased supply cost but also the allowable markup. If allowable, the hospital should use replacement cost as the base rather than actual price paid. In that way, if the price of a supply for which the hospital normally maintains a three-month inventory is increased, the price to the patient is increased immediately rather than three months later, after all of the inventory on hand has been issued.

If the formula is not mandated by a third party, in addition to ensuring that patient prices are increased as quickly as possible after a cost increase, the hospital must review the formula at least once per year. The purpose of this review is to make sure that the formula used in pricing provides enough net revenue to cover direct cost, indirect cost, and a reasonable markup on cost.

It is generally advantageous to the hospital to have pharmacy and central supply items priced according to formula. This is especially true in inflationary times because it provides for an immediate price increase that includes the cost of the item as well as an increase in total dollars of markup.

Pricing New Procedures

Throughout the year, departments initiate new services, new procedures, and new tests. A formal procedure is needed to determine the total cost of these services, procedures, and tests. This cost is then used as the basis for determining the new patient charge.

The charge for a new patient service must be high enough to cover adequately five costs: direct costs to perform the test, indirect departmental cost, the applicable portion of departmental overhead, allowances and adjustments, and reasonable markup. It is important to estimate each of these as accurately as possible because the initial charge is normally used as the basis for price increases over several years.

Direct test costs can be categorized as salary and nonsalary. To estimate salary costs, the accountant multiplies the average number of minutes it takes to perform the test by a productive costing rate for the person performing the test. The average number of minutes needed to perform the test includes set-up time, the time needed to perform the test, and clean-up time which includes returning all equipment and materials to their proper areas. It also includes the time required either to go to the patient and back or to bring the patient to and from the testing site. Often more than one employee will be involved, and average minutes required and the productive costing rate must be calculated for each employee. The productive costing rate is the average hourly pay rate for the person, inflated for nonproductive time for fringe benefits and for taxes. Nonproductive time includes holidays, vacations, sick-leave days, other paid days off, breaks, dinner hours, time away from the work station for personal needs, and an allowance for conversing with fellow employees. Average annual hours of paid days off, scheduled breaks, and dinner hours can be estimated by reviewing the personnel policies for the hospital. An allowance for other nonproductive time must be estimated after talking with department heads as well as by observing the employees. Fringe benefits and taxes are normally estimated as a percentage of total hospital payroll and applied as a percentage of payroll. Nonsalary costs to perform a test include an estimate of variable supplies.

Indirect departmental overhead includes supervision, office supplies, depreciation, maintenance and repairs, and other departmental costs. Indirect departmental overhead is calculated for each department after a careful analysis of each classification of expense for that department. This will be an estimate. Many accountants are uncomfortable with amounts that cannot be proven. However, it should be remembered that an estimate, no matter how weak, is still better than nothing.

By adding direct and indirect departmental costs together, the total departmental cost to perform the test can be determined. Applicable departmental overhead must be added to this amount. The overhead rate for each revenue-producing department can be easily determined by examining the latest step-down in which nonrevenue departments were allocated to the revenue-producing cost centers. Allowances, adjustments, and reasonable markup for each department were calculated in the pricing strategy at the beginning of the fiscal year. These same percentages can be used throughout the budget period.

The chief financial officer of the hospital should design a standard format for determining the price of new procedures. Techniques and procedures for estimating the components of cost described in this section can be found in most good cost accounting texts. It should be noted that our purpose here was to present an overview of the necessary cost accounting; our examination should not be considered a complete treatment of the subject.

Other Revenue

Other revenue includes cafeteria revenue, vending machine revenue, coffee shop revenue, television rentals, telephone rebates, purchase discounts, grants, donations, fund drives, medical records fees, silver recovery, tuitions, earned interest, and other nonpatient care revenue. For most hospitals, nonpatient revenue as a percentage of total revenue is small.

The most common method used for forecasting other revenue is to take recent historical amounts, add an appropriate inflation factor, and, if applicable, add a percentage for total utilization. It is important to have a separate general ledger account for as many other revenue accounts as practical. This allows the chief financial officer to study emerging trends. This also serves as a useful tool for internal control.

SUMMARY

Statistical budgets are the foundation upon which revenue budgets are built. If the statistics are weak, the revenue budgets will also be weak. The most critical statistic is patient days. Other statistics are either tied to or are subordinate to patient days. Patient days are forecasted in several tiers or steps. These are in total, by type of service, by month, and finally by nursing station.

There are four major types of outpatient occasions of service to consider:

1. emergency room patients who are admitted
2. emergency room patients who are ambulatory
3. referred outpatients
4. clinic visits.

Although many hospitals do not have clinic visits, most acute-care hospitals have the first three types of outpatients. To project outpatient occasions of service, the hospital uses a methodology that is similar to the one used to project inpatient days. Historical data are studied in conjunction with known or expected changes in the medical staff, in new technology, in medical economics, or from other influences.

The primary statistics are patient days and outpatient occasions of service. Once these have been projected, the ancillary services, which are secondary or dependent statistics, can be forecasted. There are several methods that have been used successfully to project ancillary service statistics. The important point to remember is that ancillary department heads should participate in forecasting workloads for their departments.

Budgeting revenue in hospitals is the mechanical process of taking the hospital's targeted net gain, adding expected expenses to arrive at targeted revenue, adding allowances and adjustments to arrive at targeted gross revenue, and finally raising prices enough to meet gross revenue. Expected gain is the amount needed to stay solvent, provide for new technology, provide for physical plant renovation or replacement, and provide for increased working capital needs. Forecasted expenses are the amounts projected in the hospital's expense budget. Allowances and adjustments include bad debts, free care, charity, contractual adjustments for cost reports, other contractual adjustments, discounts, and other revenue deductions.

Before the hospital raises prices, it should have a well-defined pricing strategy. There are three components of a good pricing strategy: average price increase, departmental price increase, and individual-procedure price increase. Price increases result in additional net revenue only from billed-charge paying patients. Patient care that is reimbursed on a cost contract is not affected by price increases. The purpose of pricing strategy is to increase net revenue by reducing contractual allowances. A key tool in setting prices is a departmental ranking schedule that identifies by department the percentage of charge-based revenue and the percentage of cost-based revenue.

The charge for a new patient service must be high enough to cover direct cost to perform the test and also indirect departmental cost. In addition to these departmental costs, the charge must cover institutional costs, such as overhead allocated to the department, allowances and adjustments, and a reasonable markup.

DISCUSSION QUESTIONS

1. Identify the three steps in a statistical budget for patient days.
2. Define the four types of outpatient occasions of service.
3. Explain the three components that make up budgeted revenue.
4. Identify the various components that make up patient revenue from price increases.
5. What is a departmental ranking schedule? How is this used to develop a departmental pricing strategy? How is it used to develop an individual-procedure pricing strategy?
6. If pharmacy or central supply prices are based on a formula rather than a stated amount for each item, what can be done to maximize net revenue?
7. What are some of the costs that should be considered by the accountant in setting prices for a new procedure?
8. What are some of the advantages of having separate general ledger accounts for the various other revenue categories?

Chapter 8

Monthly Analysis and Reports

In Chapters 6 and 7, we examined the techniques and methodologies used to prepare the hospital's annual budget. If the hospital waited until year end to analyze the results of operations, it would be too late to take corrective action. Financial analysis must be performed monthly. In this chapter we will examine how to convert the annual budget into monthly budgets. We will also look at several monthly reports and illustrate some techniques used to analyze monthly operations.

CONVERTING ANNUAL BUDGETS TO MONTHLY BUDGETS

Before converting the annual expense budget to monthly budgets, the hospital should separate salary expenses from nonsalary expenses. Salary expenses include both payroll and applicable fringe benefits. Revenue and revenue offsets should be considered separately from expenses.

Payroll Expenses

There are several techniques that can be used to produce accurate monthly payroll-expense forecasts. The actual technique used will depend upon the data base available as well as the personal preference of the chief financial officer.

A good monthly position control that budgets hours by department should be used as the basis for the salary expense budget. The department develops an average pay rate for the year by dividing budgeted salary expense by budgeted hours. This average departmental pay rate is converted to a monthly average pay rate. The monthly pay rate takes into account annual employee pay increases, high overtime months, and, if appropriate, high vacation-usage months. The monthly average pay rate is multiplied by the budgeted hours for each month. The 12 calculated salary expense amounts are then totaled and compared to the annual budgeted amount. If the difference is insignificant, the calculated amounts can be adjusted so that the total of the 12 salary expense amounts is equal to the annual forecast. If the difference is substantial, the assumptions and statistics supporting the annual budget figure are compared to the assumptions and statistics used to support the individual monthly figures. The total of the monthly amounts must equal the annual salary budget for each department.

Another effective technique used to convert the annual departmental salary budget into monthly budgets is to develop a salary distribution schedule. This schedule will determine the percentage of annual salary to distribute to each month. A departmental distribution schedule is calculated by taking the salary expense for each month of the last fiscal year and dividing these amounts by the total annual salary. For example, assume a department had $10,000 of salary expense in January of last year and $140,000 of salary expense for that year.

The percentage of salary for January is 10 divided by 140, or 7.14 percent. In this year's budget, the month of January would be allocated 7.14 percent of the total salary expense. This calculation would be performed for each month of the fiscal year until the entire salary expense budget for each department is divided into 12 monthly amounts.

The hospital can increase the accuracy of the salary distribution schedules by taking a weighted average of several years' monthly percentages by department. By weighting recent years more heavily than prior years, the hospital will be budgeting the most recent payroll distribution trends and at the same time will partially negate any unusual factors and circumstances that may distort any single year.

Once salary expense by department by month has been forecasted, the hospital should distribute annual fringe-benefit expense to each of the 12 months. If the hospital has budgeted sick pay, vacation pay, holidays, jury duty, bereavement pay, and other nonproductive salary expenses as fringe benefits, these amounts must be separated from other fringe benefits and allocated to the 12 months using the same methodology as that used for salary expense. Social Security, workmen's compensation, federal and state unemployment compensation, life insurance, health insurance, executive perquisites, and other fringe benefits should be calculated as a percentage of salary expense by department. If the hospital budgets nonproductive salary expense as a fringe benefit, this should be reclassified to salary expense before calculating the fringe-benefit percentage. This percentage is used to spread fringe benefits by department to the 12 months.

It is important to calculate the fringe-benefit percentage separately for each department. Many hospitals charge some benefits to an administrative account rather than to the departments. For example, in many hospitals workmen's compensation, unemployment compensation, and life insurance are charged to administration. By calculating a fringe-benefit percentage separately for each department, the amount budgeted each month will reflect the hospital's accounting treatment of fringe benefits. This will make variance analysis more meaningful throughout the budget period.

Nonpayroll Expenses

Significant nonpayroll expenses that can be easily identified should be identified and budgeted separately by month. The expenses to be identified and the manner in which they are budgeted monthly should be determined after studying the hospital's accounting practices. This will reduce budget variances throughout the forecast period. If interest expense is expensed when paid, this should be budgeted in the months in which interest payments are due. If interest expense is accrued on a monthly basis, the expense should be budgeted in 12 equal amounts.

Other expenses that are often budgeted separately on a monthly basis include utilities, insurance, depreciation, service contracts, telephone expense, and amortization expense. It must be cautioned that the manner in which these expenses are budgeted must be exactly the same as the manner in which the hospital's accounting practices expense them. Otherwise, variance analysis on a monthly basis will not be meaningful.

Once the chief financial officer has identified those significant expenses that should be budgeted using a separate analysis, the remaining annual expenses must be allocated to the 12 months. One way to accomplish this is to calculate by month and by department the percentage of these expenses in the last completed fiscal year. This technique was explained earlier in the section on payroll expenses. The percentages can be refined by taking a weighted average of several years. The percentage by month can then be used to allocate the annual expenses to the 12 months for the budget period.

A more accurate technique is to develop a budget distribution schedule. This schedule will define parameters that will determine the final distribution by period of the proposed budget for all general ledger accounts. Table 8–1 is a sample budget distribution schedule for Community Hospital.

This budget distribution schedule should be considered only as a guide. The statistics shown do not represent an all-inclusive list of possible distribution statistics, nor will these statistics be applicable to all hospitals. The logic used to distribute annual budget amounts should be determined by each hospital to reflect its individual needs.

Using the budget distribution schedule, the hospital should determine on an individual basis the statistic used to allocate in monthly increments the annual budgeted amount for each remaining general ledger amount. The monthly budgets are then summarized and presented to department heads in the same format that will be used for their monthly actual-expense reports.

Table 8–1 Community Hospital Budget Distribution Schedule

Year Ended December 31, 19X0

Total	January	February	March	December	Statistic
		Percentage by Period			
100.0	9.00	8.00	8.45 . . . . 7.55		Patient day forecast
100.0	8.30	8.20	8.25 . . . . 8.26		Outpatient occasions
100.0	8.95	8.05	8.30 . . . . 7.68		Adjusted patient days
100.0	8.49	7.67	8.49 . . . . 8.49		Calendar days
100.0	8.81	7.66	8.05 . . . . 8.81		Number of weekdays
100.0	8.41	7.90	8.45 . . . . 8.50		Budget payroll expense
100.0	8.33	8.33	8.33 . . . . 8.33		Equal monthly amount

Revenue and Revenue Offsets

The annual revenue budgets were based upon the hospital statistical budget. These same budgetary statistics are used to convert the annual gross revenue amounts to monthly revenue budgets. In finalizing the monthly gross revenue budgets, the accountant must make sure that any price increases are accounted for. If the hospital increases prices only at the beginning of its fiscal year, the only price increases that need to be separately calculated by month are those which are based upon a formula. In the previous chapter, we saw that prices for the pharmacy and central-supply items are often determined by a formula based upon hospital costs. In these cases, the average revenue per occasion of service or per patient day will increase throughout the year as charges to the patient reflect higher costs paid to suppliers.

Revenue deductions include bad debts, charity, contractual adjustment discounts, and allowances. Except for contractual adjustments, these offsets as a percentage of gross revenue do not normally vary significantly from month to month. Contractual adjustments are a function of the difference between billed charges and allowable costs. Prices remain relatively stable throughout the year, while costs increase with inflation. The difference between billed charges and allowable costs, therefore, is greater in the early months of the fiscal year and less acute in the later months of the fiscal year. If the hospital's accounting is sophisticated enough to measure and record this difference, the budget should reflect it. For all other revenue deductions, as well as for contractual adjustments that are not tracked on a monthly basis, the hospital should calculate a percentage of gross revenue and use this percentage to allocate deductions to the 12 months.

Other revenue is normally not significant in most hospitals. This revenue includes cafeteria income, vending machine and telephone rebates, tuition, rentals, and other income. This revenue is normally allocated 1/12th to each month.

Considerations

The usefulness of the budget versus actual reports is directly proportional to the quality of the techniques used to convert the annual budget to monthly budgets. If expense or revenue items are significantly offbudget at the end of the first quarter, the hospital will normally take corrective action of some kind. Therefore, it is important that this variance be real rather than the result of a budget timing error. If these monthly budgets are accurate, decisions to act upon budget variances can be made with confidence. If the monthly budgets are mediocre, only mediocre decisions can be made based upon budget variances. If the monthly budgets merely show 1/12th of the annual budget for each category and are not properly adjusted for seasonal variations, they are almost meaningless. The time spent converting the annual budget to monthly budgets will be rewarded 12 times in the coming year.

The budget figures when presented should never be broken down beyond the nearest whole dollar and should seldom be broken down beyond the nearest ten dollars by month. Large amounts should be rounded to the nearest one hundred dollars. When budgets that are not rounded off are presented to department heads, there is an implied accuracy that does not, in fact, exist. This implied accuracy often motivates department heads to use the budget as a target to be met at all costs rather than as a management tool. Budgets that have been rounded off are a more useful management tool.

Often the sum of the 12 monthly budgets will not equal the annual budget. This is because of rounding errors in conversion. This can be prevented if the person filling out the worksheets balances the monthly totals to the annual amounts on an account-by-account basis. The amount of the variance for any account will be small. One or two months can be arbitrarily adjusted to force the monthly budgets to equal the annual amount.

MONTHLY REPORTS

In this section we will describe a series of monthly reports used by hospitals to monitor financial progress, spending patterns, and management efficiency. The list does not include all possible management reports. However, our discussion will be comprehensive enough to give the reader a good understanding of the kinds of information needed to make informed decisions.

Comparisons of Actual to Budget

Every hospital should have a minimum of four sets of monthly reports comparing actual to budget. These are departmental reports, program reports, the hospital statement of income and expense, and sources of applications of cash.

Most departmental reports show actual, budget, and variance for both the current period and the fiscal year to date. These reports are used by department managers in controlling direct costs. An example of a departmental report for the outpatient clinic of a typical hospital is shown in Table 8–2.

The title of the sample report shows both the name of the cost center and the general ledger account number. If the hospital assigns a different account number for revenue and for expense, the expense number should show on the budget report. The name of the department manager, D. Smith, is also shown on this report.

Each budgeted departmental account should be detailed separately on the department budget reports. Revenue-producing departments should be held accountable for budgeting revenue as well as for explaining budget variances. The

Table 8-2 A Departmental Report for an Outpatient Clinic

Department 200—Outpatient Clinic

D. Smith

Account	Description	Current Month			Year to Date		
		Actual	Budget	Variance	Actual	Budget	Variance
050	Clinic	XXX	XXX	XX	XXX	XXX	XX
060	Prof. fees	XXX	XXX	XX	XXX	XXX	XX
Total revenue		XXX	XXX	XX	XXX	XXX	XX
100	Salaries-prof.	XXX	XXX	XX	XXX	XXX	XX
150	Salaries-nursing	XXX	XXX	XX	XXX	XXX	XX
170	Salaries-other	XXX	XXX	XX	XXX	XXX	XX
200	Social security	XXX	XXX	XX	XXX	XXX	XX
210	Health insurance	XXX	XXX	XX	XXX	XXX	XX
Total personnel expense		XXX	XXX	XX	XXX	XXX	XX
310	Drugs	XXX	XXX	XX	XXX	XXX	XX
320	Medical supplies	XXX	XXX	XX	XXX	XXX	XX
330	Other supplies	XXX	XXX	XX	XXX	XXX	XX
410	Service contracts	XXX	XXX	XX	XXX	XXX	XX
420	Repairs-maintenance	XXX	XXX	XX	XXX	XXX	XX
500	Travel	XXX	XXX	XX	XXX	XXX	XX
600	Miscellaneous expense	XXX	XXX	XX	XXX	XXX	XX
Total nonpersonnel expense		XXX	XXX	XX	XXX	XXX	XX
Total expense		XXX	XXX	XX	XXX	XXX	XX
Net gain (loss)		XXX	XXX	XX	XXX	XXX	XX

example shown in Table 8–2 reports revenue on the same page with expenses. Many hospitals report revenue separately by department. Although the department heads have limited control over revenue, there are two important reasons why they should be required to explain significant budget variances. First, if department heads are managing their revenue, problems with lost charges, missing charges, price increases, and other factors that prohibit the hospital from maximizing gross revenue are placed at the level of responsibility where timely corrective action can be taken. Second, if department heads are managing their revenue, the hospital will have a more accurate annual revenue forecast. In addition to reports expressed in whole dollars, it is useful to give department managers reports that compare budgeted statistics with actual and budgeted unit cost to actual. Table 8–3 is an example of a format used to report statistics and unit costs for an outpatient clinic. Unlike the whole dollar reports, unit cost statistics should be reported in summary form.

Program reports should show the same detail and be in the same format as department reports. These programs can be prepared either by reporting responsibility or by function. If reporting responsibility is used, all cost centers that report to the director of nursing would summarize in one report, all cost centers that report to an assistant administrator would summarize in another report, and so on. If the program reports summarize by function, all ancillaries would be on one page, all inpatient nursing units on another page, all outpatient nursing units on a third page, and so on.

The hospital statement of income and expense should be presented with a comparison to budget. This comparison should compare actual results to budget for every line on the hospital's regular income statement. It is especially useful to report the total hospital income statement in both whole dollars and per unit cost. The unit costs most often used are inpatient days and adjusted patient days. Adjusted patient days are equal to inpatient days plus outpatient activity expressed as equivalent patient days. Adjusted patient days can be calculated by using the following formula:

$$\text{Patient Days} \times \frac{\text{Inpatient Revenue} + \text{Outpatient Revenue}}{\text{Inpatient Revenue}} = \begin{array}{l}\text{Adjusted}\\\text{Patient}\\\text{Days}\end{array}$$

Some hospitals have developed an extensive income and expense budget reporting system but have failed to report the budget versus actual cash position by month. Often the controller fails to report the ending cash balance each month. It must be remembered that all purchases, liabilities, and expenses are paid out of cash. Therefore, it is important that the hospital prepare a detailed comparison of actual to budget sources and the application of cash every month. The preparation of a cash budget is covered in a later chapter.

Although the formats shown in this section are the most common, many hospitals successfully use comparisons of actual to budget in different formats.

Table 8-3 Format for Reporting Statistics and Unit Costs

Department 200—Outpatient Clinic

D. Smith

| Description | Current Month | | | Year to Date | | |
	Actual	Budget	Variance	Actual	Budget	Variance
Clinic visits	XXX	XXX	XX	XXX	XXX	XX
Per clinic visit						
Revenue	XXX	XXX	XX	XXX	XXX	XX
Salary expense	XXX	XXX	XX	XXX	XXX	XX
Supply expense	XXX	XXX	XX	XXX	XXX	XX
Other expense	XXX	XXX	XX	XXX	XXX	XX
Net gain (loss)	XXX	XXX	XX	XXX	XXX	XX

As an example, some hospitals compare actual results to prior year's results as well as to budget. Some reports show actual and either budget or variance accounts but not both. The actual format used should be one that the department heads and the administrator feel is most effective.

Supporting Schedules

In addition to the four sets of monthly reports described in the previous section, many hospitals prepare supporting schedules that track special problem areas or report other information used by administration. In this section we will list or describe some of the most common supporting schedules used by hospitals.

The month-end balance sheet is sometimes compared to the beginning of the period with a column titled net change. For example, a balance sheet may report six columns of information. For the current month, it would show beginning of period, end of period, and either net change or percentage change for each item on the balance sheet. The report would also show beginning of period, end of period, and either net change or percentage change for the year to date.

Most hospitals that prepare supporting schedules will have at least one schedule to analyze revenue. For each revenue-producing department, revenue can be shown broken down into outpatient and inpatient, with that particular department shown as a percentage of the total. Table 8–4 is an example of a supporting schedule for revenue.

This schedule could show revenue per patient day or per adjusted patient day rather than by each department's percentage of the total. Additional reports on the following revenue areas can be generated if the hospital has electronic data processing: total revenue by admitting physician, total revenue by nursing unit or by floor, total revenue by medical specialty, average revenue per admission or per day by admitting physician or by admitting diagnosis, and total revenue by procedure or test for the period. With electronic data processing, supporting schedules are limited only by the amount of accurate source-document information and the technical capability of the data-processing staff.

Table 8–4 Community Hospital—Supporting Schedule for Revenue

Department	Inpatient		Outpatient		Total	
	Amount	%	Amount	%	Amount	%
Routine services	XXX	XX	XXX	XX	XXX	XX
Laboratory	XXX	XX	XXX	XX	XXX	XX
	↓	↓	↓	↓	↓	↓
Total	XXX	100%	XXX	100%	XXX	100%

Supplies expense by department and professional fees by department are frequently used to monitor these high-dollar expenditures. Other monthly supporting schedules may include deductions from revenue, other revenue, and drug expense by department. If the hospital has a program to allocate nonrevenue-producing departments to revenue-producing departments, several performance analysis reports can be generated that will quickly identify areas needing special management attention in order to maximize third party reimbursement. A departmental performance analysis report shows gross revenue reduced by allowances and deductions, direct expense, and allocated indirect expense to arrive at an actual gain or loss. The two most common methods of allocating indirect cost (nonrevenue-producing departments) to the revenue-producing departments are stepdown and simultaneous equations.

The many different supporting schedules we have described provide a basis for developing many more schedules. Hospital administrators should develop an intuitive or acquired ability to determine the cost-benefit ratio of all new reports as well as ongoing reports. They need to ask if this report is worth the time and expense it will take to develop and maintain it. Will the users of the report be able to absorb and use all of the information, or would a simpler, less expensive report be just as beneficial? If the schedule does not pass this cost-benefit analysis test, it should not be prepared.

Statistical Budget Reports

In addition to supporting income and expense schedules, many hospitals find it helpful to report budgeted operating indicators. This includes the number of admissions, patient days, outpatient occasions of service, tests or procedures by department, man-hours by department, and other statistics. Operating or workload statistics can be effectively presented in graph or table form. It is especially useful to prepare a graph to illustrate a trend or trends covering several years.

For department managers, statistical budget comparisons are a more effective tool than actual dollar comparisons. An example of a statistical budget comparison for the radiology department of Community Hospital is shown in Table 8–5.

This example not only shows hours worked but also hours worked per procedure and nonproductive hours. Statistical budgets that break costs, hours, or other statistics down to a workload basis are much more effective than budgets that report unadjusted statistics. This is because it is easy to relate to a procedure, a patient day, or a test but difficult to relate to hundreds of procedures, patient days, or tests. Time spent breaking statistical budgets down to a lower common denominator is normally effective.

The example shown in Table 8–5 reports nonproductive hours. These include vacation, sick-leave days, holidays, jury duty, and other time in which the

Table 8–5 Community Hospital—Radiology Statistical Budget

	Current Month		Year to Date	
	Bud	Act	Bud	Act
Productive hours	1,300	1,183	4,400	4,375
Per procedure	.52	.61	.52	.47
Nonproductive hours	20	29	100	294
Total hours	1,320	1,212	4,500	4,669
Average hourly rate	5.55	5.30	5.55	5.33
Per procedure	2.30	2.60	2.30	2.53
Number of procedures	2,500	1,939	8,461	9,309
Hospital patient days	6,200	6,000	31,000	33,000

employee is paid but not working. To show this on a per procedure basis would not be meaningful. The statistical budget also shows hospital patient days in order to report the general activity that affects the radiology department.

This example shows some statistics that may be useful to a radiology manager. It is not meant to be all-inclusive. Other statistics that could be considered are procedures per patient days, salary expense per procedure, nonsalary expense per procedure, and total expense per patient day. In addition to showing current month and year to date, it may be useful to report prior-year statistics, prior-month statistics, or next month's statistics. The information presented on statistical reports should be tailored to fit the needs of the individual hospital.

Variance Analysis

Monthly analysis of significant budget variances has a twofold purpose. First, it acts as a control by requiring managers to identify any potential problem areas. Potential problem areas, once identified, are further analyzed. Second, the reports represent a historical account of whatever creates a significant unfavorable variance. Managers as well as administration become very knowledgeable about the major spending patterns within the institution.

The hospital should have definite policies to determine responsibility for analysis-of-budget variances. The responsibility can either be centralized in the accounting department or the departments can be required to analyze and report their own variances. If the accounting department prepares the variance analysis for all departments, department heads should participate in explaining major variances to the accounting analyst. It is important to have the department heads involved as much as possible in studying budget variances.

Identification of budget variances to report each month is a judgmental matter to be decided by each hospital. In establishing parameters, the hospital should remember that one of the purposes of this report is to provide a historical account of spending patterns. It is better to have too much detail than not enough. The following can be used as a guide:

- Seldom are variances of less than one hundred dollars significant.

- The expense should be reasonable for the function of the particular department. For example, accounting should never report research supplies or drug expense.

- If a pattern of overspending occurs each month and is explainable, it should be included only occasionally in the written variance description.

- Significant variances are a function of percentage as well as of dollar amount. For example, a variance of two hundred dollars is significant for an item budgeted at one hundred dollars for the period but is not significant for an item budgeted at one hundred thousand dollars for the period.

Miscellaneous Projects and Reports

As the reports described in this section are prepared, the controller and the administrator will become keenly aware of many financial trends and practices. The reports will provide a comprehensive understanding of financial causes and effects. Several patterns that could be potential problems will begin to develop throughout the year. These patterns should be analyzed, summarized, and presented by the controller, along with suggested courses of action where appropriate.

RATIO ANALYSIS

No monthly analysis of an entity as complicated as a modern hospital would be complete without a focus from a banker's or financial analyst's viewpoint. In using a ratio analysis, it is important to remember that a set of financial statements by itself has very little meaning. Financial statements are useful as management tools only when they are compared to something. Ratio analysis enables the user to study financial strengths and weaknesses by identifying trends. Our discussion will not consider all possible ratios, nor will it cover all the fine points in those that are mentioned. It will examine some commonly used ratios and show how these can be useful to any hospital.

Ability To Meet Current Obligations

The *current ratio* is computed by dividing the current assets by the current liabilities. If the current ratio becomes smaller over time it can be concluded that the hospital may have some difficulty in paying its bills. An unusually high or a growing current ratio suggests that the hospital may not be using funds effectively. If no better yardstick is available, a rough rule of thumb suggests that a current ratio of 2 to 1 is satisfactory. However, the movement of changes in the current ratio is more important than the numerical ratio as of any given date.

Cash to operating expenses is computed by dividing the ending cash balance by 1/12th of the annual operating expenses. Although a hospital must maintain enough cash to meet its obligations, excessive cash on hand can represent poor management. Hospitals that report this ratio should also report the number of days until the next payroll.

The *quick ratio* is computed by dividing the quick assets by the current liabilities. In most industries, the quick assets include cash marketable securities, and net receivables, but exclude inventory and prepaid expenses. In a hospital, inventories are normally short lived, but it will take a long time to realize all of the net receivables. The quick assets for a hospital would, therefore, include cash, marketable securities, and inventories but exclude net receivables and prepaid expenses. The hospital may want to examine its collection time lag and include a specified percentage of net receivables in quick assets and exclude other net receivables. The assets included in quick assets are not important as long as all readers of the ratio analysis understand what is being used. Consistency is very important, and the definition of quick assets must remain the same. In the absence of other comparative data, the minimum acceptable quick ratio for a hospital is 1 to 1.

Percentage composition of current assets is computed by taking each of the current assets as a percentage of total current assets. The further removed an asset on the balance is from cash, the less liquid it is. Percentage composition of current assets determines on a monthly basis what percentage of the current assets is in the form of cash, what percentage is one step removed (accounts receivable), and what percentage is two steps removed (inventory).

Effective Use of Assets

The *average collection period* or *number of days in receivables* can be calculated on either a monthly or an annualized basis. The formulas are as follows.

Monthly Basis:
$$\frac{\text{Accounts Receivable} \times \text{Days in Month}}{\text{Monthly Net Income}} = \text{Days in Receivables}$$

Annualized Basis:
$$\frac{\text{Accounts Receivable} \times 365}{\text{Annualized Net Income}} = \text{Days in Receivables}$$

An alternative method that provides the same kind of management information is to determine the receivables turnover. Receivables turnover is computed by dividing annualized net income by accounts receivable or monthly net income, times 12, divided by accounts receivable. If the annual rate of turnover is 6, this means that, on the average, receivables are collected in 2 months. If the turnover rate is 4, then on the average receivables are collected in 3 months.

The reason for using days in receivables as well as receivables turnover is to measure the liquidity of the accounts receivables. This is important for two reasons. The longer funds remain in accounts receivable, the longer the hospital must forego use of this cash. Even more important is the fact that the older an account gets, the less likely it is to become fully collected.

Inventory turnover is computed by dividing supply expense by average inventory. This ratio can be calculated separately for central supply, for pharmacy, for dietary, and for general stores. It can also be calculated in total for the entire hospital. Within limits, the higher the inventory turnover the better. Inventory management is a compromise between being out of stock on occasion and tying up funds in inventory.

Other ratios that have been used to measure the effective use of assets include net revenue to net working capital and net revenue to fund balance. Net revenue to net working capital measures the adequacy of working capital to support the patient revenue. As revenue increases over time, working capital should increase proportionately. Net revenue to fund balance measures the amount of fund balance that supports the current patient revenue level.

Adequacy of Net Gain

Are the earnings or net gain adequate? This is a crucial question for management because it relates to the long-term financial viability or stability of the hospital.

Times interest earned is computed by dividing the net gain before interest (if a for-profit hospital, before taxes) by annual interest charges. The interest coverage is especially important in hospitals because of the large portion of third-party cost reimbursement. Cost reimbursement creates a situation where budget variances have a more pronounced effect on net gain.

Rate of earnings on total assets employed is calculated by dividing net gain before interest (if a for-profit hospital, before taxes) by total assets. This ratio is a measure of the hospital's earning power on total assets. A similar ratio might be calculated to measure rate of return on total assets employed for each revenue-producing department. This would be especially useful to measure in the large ancillary departments.

Net gain to total expenses is total net gain divided by total expenses. This measures the effectiveness of the hospital's pricing strategy as well as the quality of third-party cost report preparation.

Net gain to fund balance divides the final net gain by final fund balance. This measures the amount of total accumulated fund balance that was contributed in the current period.

Distribution of Assets

Net receivables to net working capital is computed by dividing ending net receivables by net working capital. Working capital is defined as total current assets minus total current liabilities. Net receivables are normally the largest item in current assets and consequently the greatest portion of net working capital. The higher the net receivables as a percentage of working capital, the greater the possibility of getting into financial difficulty if the patient census should decline suddenly.

Fixed assets to fund balance is total net fixed assets divided by fund balance. The more a hospital has invested in fixed assets, the less flexible it can be in its operations. If this ratio becomes greater over time, the hospital should consider leasing instead of purchasing new equipment until fund balance increases substantially.

Use of Ratios

The use of ratio analysis has been a common practice in industry for many years. Bankers, investment analysts, and others have also used ratios to study the financial direction of borrowers. Ratio analysis has not been widely used in hospitals in the past. However, with today's growing financial pressures, more hospitals are using this powerful management tool.

The number of ratios that might be utilized in studying financial statements is almost limitless. Each hospital will have its preferences. The chief financial officer and chief executive officer should decide what kinds of trends need to be followed and then choose ratios that will give the desired information. All hospitals should calculate at least four ratios on a monthly basis. One should measure the hospital's ability to meet current obligations. Others should measure the effective use of assets, the adequacy of earnings, and the distribution of assets. Most hospitals should calculate more than four ratios monthly.

The calculation of ratios is a simple mathematical process. Their interpretation, however, requires some basis for comparison. The most useful comparisons are those that compare identical ratios for the same enterprise over different time periods. There is no better way to track the financial direction for a hospital or any other enterprise.

SUMMARY

The first step in converting annual expense budgets to monthly budgets is to separate nonsalary expenses from payroll expenses and fringe benefits. Techniques used successfully to prepare monthly payroll forecasts include multiplying average departmental pay rates by monthly position control hours if available and developing a salary distribution schedule based upon monthly historical salary-expense patterns. Average departmental pay rates can vary significantly from month to month because of pay increases, high overtime months, and high vacation-usage months. The accuracy of a salary distribution schedule can be increased by taking a weighted average of several years' monthly percentages by department.

If the hospital has budgeted nonproductive salary expense as a fringe benefit, these amounts must be separated from other fringe benefits and allocated to the 12 months using the same methodology that is used for salary expense. Other fringe benefits should be calculated as a percentage of salary expense by department. The departmental fringe-benefit percentage must be calculated separately for each hospital department.

Significant nonsalary expenses that can be easily identified are culled out and budgeted separately. Other nonsalary expenses are distributed using historical spending patterns or by developing a budget distribution schedule. Revenue budgets are based on statistical workload forecasts.

Every hospital should have four sets of monthly reports comparing actual to budget. These are departmental reports, program reports, hospital statement of income and expense, and sources and applications of cash. These reports normally show actual, budget, and variance for both the current period and the fiscal year to date. The departmental reports should show as much detail as the annual budget. Program reports summarize some expense categories.

Supporting schedules track special problem areas or report other information that is used by administration. These schedules are different for every hospital. Most hospitals that use supporting schedules have at least one to analyze revenue. Before initiating a new supporting schedule, administration should subject it to a cost-benefit ratio test.

Financial statements are useful as management tools only when they are compared to something. Ratio analysis enables the user to study financial strengths and weaknesses by identifying trends. Ratio analysis is used to judge the hospital's ability to meet current obligations, to measure the effective use of assets, to measure the adequacy of net gain, to test the distribution of assets, and for other purposes. There is no better way to track the financial direction of a hospital than to use a comparative ratio analysis over different time periods.

DISCUSSION QUESTIONS

1. Explain two methodologies that can be used to convert annual salary budgets to monthly salary budgets.
2. What is a budget distribution schedule? How is it used?
3. Why is it important to convert annual budgets to monthly budgets in an accurate, well-defined manner?
4. What are the four most important sets of monthly budget comparisons used by hospitals?
5. Explain the advantages to be gained by requiring revenue department heads to manage their own revenue budgets, including the use of variance analysis.
6. Define adjusted patient days.
7. Describe a specific supporting schedule and explain how it would be used by you if you were a hospital administrator.
8. How are monthly variance analyses used?
9. What is the difference between computing number of days in receivables and receivables turnover?
10. Explain one ratio used to measure distribution of assets.
11. What is the purpose of performing a monthly ratio analysis?

Chapter 9

Cost Reimbursement

Cost-based reimbursement accounts for a larger portion of hospital revenue every year. As cost reimbursement continues to grow, it will become more important for every member of hospital management to understand how cost-based reimbursement works. In this chapter we will explain the major principles and concepts of cost-based reimbursement in nontechnical language. We will also outline some techniques that can be used to maximize cost reimbursement.

OVERVIEW OF PRINCIPLES

In this section we will use illustrations to show how hospital costs are reimbursed.

Container of Costs

Assume that all of the costs necessary to operate the hospital are in a container, as in Figure 9–1. Each year more costs are added to the container. In the past, approximately two-thirds of the increase in hospital costs each year was due to inflation. Inflation affects salary rates, taxes, fringe benefits, increases in prices for supplies, utilities, services, and other prices. Inflationary increases are called normal because they are common to all industries. Approximately one-third of the increase in hospital costs each year has historically been due to new and better services. This includes increases in the number of tests performed per patient day, new procedures, new drugs, technology that is new to the hospital, and average salary rate increases that are due to the need for higher skill levels.

Another way to describe new and better cost increases is to talk about patient acuity. Every hospital is saving lives of people who would have died a few years ago. Every hospital is dispensing drugs that were not available a few years ago. Every hospital has more sophisticated diagnostic and treatment equipment

Figure 9–1 Container of Costs Needed To Run a Hospital

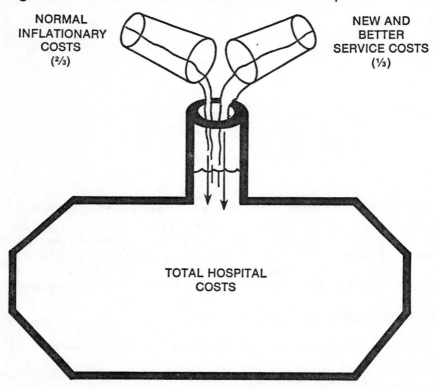

NORMAL
INFLATIONARY
COSTS
(⅔)

NEW AND
BETTER
SERVICE COSTS
(⅓)

TOTAL HOSPITAL
COSTS

than it did a few years ago. Patient acuity must be measured for each hospital individually. It makes no difference how long a procedure or a piece of equipment has been used by other hospitals in the area. The first year the procedure or the equipment is available in a particular hospital, it increases the technology available to serve that hospital's patients. A more acute illness can now be successfully diagnosed or treated by that hospital. Therefore, the costs to provide that new service are new and better costs.

In our example, if costs were to increase by $15 per patient day, we would know that $10 was due to inflation and $5 due to providing new and better services.

Distribution of Cost Increases

Now let us see how these costs are absorbed. Let us assume that our container is equipped with a standpipe to absorb the increases in costs which the hospital must incur. The container with standpipes is shown in Figure 9–2.

Figure 9–2 Container of Hospital Costs with Cost-absorbing Standpipes

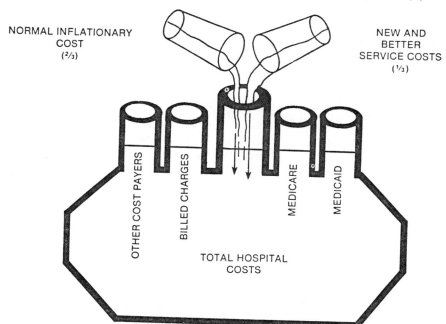

NORMAL INFLATIONARY
COST
(^{2}/$_3$)

NEW AND
BETTER
SERVICE COSTS
(^{1}/$_3$)

OTHER COST PAYERS

BILLED CHARGES

MEDICARE

MEDICAID

TOTAL HOSPITAL
COSTS

There is a standpipe for billed-charges payers, for Medicare, for Medicaid, and for other cost payers. Other cost payers include all non-Medicare and non-Medicaid payers who reimburse the hospital on a basis other than billed charges. This includes Blue Cross in those states where Blue Cross reimburses on a cost report. It also includes costs covered by special agreements with health maintenance organizations, social agencies, government programs that pay on a per-diem basis regardless of how that per diem is computed, contracts with other providers, and other programs that do not pay billed charges. Billed charges include costs covered by a payer whose payments are based on the hospital's actual billed charges. This includes most commercial insurance companies, patients who pay all or part of their charges, some social agencies, and others. Billed charges do not include amounts for bad debts, charity, contractual adjustments, and other deductions from revenue. The hospital cannot pass cost increases on to patients who do not pay. Medicare and Medicaid includes only that portion of the patient's charges that is covered by the applicable program. Patient coinsurance and deductible amounts are included in the standpipe for billed charges.

In physics we are taught that fluids, if not constrained, will seek their own level. In our example, we would expect other cost payers, billed charges, Medicare, and Medicaid to absorb a proportionate share of cost increases every year. We would also expect each standpipe to absorb a proportionate share of the cost of providing hospital service to charity, bad debt, and other classes of patients that do not pay. If there were no artificial constraints and hospitals were allowed to charge all patients equally, this would happen. However, certain payers impose limits upon the amount of cost increases they will absorb.

Cost-Based Third Party Payers

Medicare, Medicaid, and other payers that do not pay billed charges in effect constrain the amount of costs that they will absorb. These constraints are represented by stopcocks in Figure 9–3.

By releasing pressure on the stopcock in its standpipe, a cost payer absorbs a portion of the hospital's cost increases. By freezing the position of their stopcock, the cost payers freeze revenue per patient day for patients covered under their programs; and, by screwing the stopcock down, cost payers can, in effect, pass part of the cost that is appropriately theirs on to other patients. In

Figure 9–3 Container of Hospital Costs with Stopcock Constraints on Cost-Absorbing Standpipes

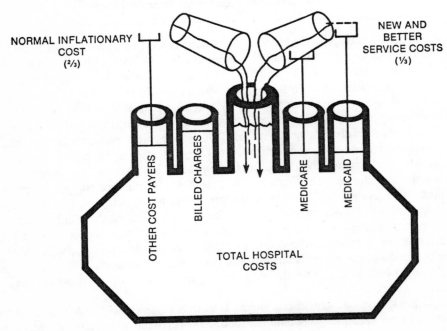

our example, there is a dotted line connecting the Medicare and the Medicaid stopcock handles. This is because Medicaid reimbursement is dependent upon Medicare reimbursement. The hospital completes its Medicare cost report first. The Medicaid cost report for each state is designed individually. However, Medicaid reimbursement is based on Medicare principles, and the instructions to complete a significant portion of the Medicaid cost report normally refer to lines on one of the Medicare schedules.

In the past, Medicare and Medicaid have absorbed only a fraction of their applicable cost increases. The government acknowledges an obligation to pay for normal cost increases but not for any of the cost increases associated with providing new and better services. Other cost-based payers have generally raised the stopcock enough each year to absorb their portion of cost increases, but no more. It is important to remember that as long as a payer does not reimburse based on billed charges, there is a chance that the stopcock will not be raised enough to absorb all applicable costs.

It should be obvious from the above discussion that hospitals have been forced to raise prices a disproportionate amount in order to cover costs. This in turn has forced billed-charges payers to absorb a disproportionate share of health care costs. As the fluid in the billed charges pipe rises to the brim, it reaches a spillover point. The spillover point is that economic point where patients, insurance companies, social agencies, and others in this category either cannot or will not pay the hospital's published charges. This spillover point is shown in Figure 9–4. If the hospital is in a state in which Blue Cross reimburses on a cost contract, Blue Cross will have a distinct and measurable price advantage over other health insurance companies.

The Cost Dilemma

It should be clear from the above discussion that hospital price increases generally affect only that class of patients who pay billed charges. To illustrate, assume Hospital A is 50-percent cost reimbursed and Hospital B is 70-percent cost reimbursed. Both hospitals experience a 5-percent charity and bad debt rate. Assume further that average charges per patient day are $200 at each hospital, average reimbursable cost is $180, and both hospitals initiate a 10-percent price increase. The effect of this price increase is shown in Table 9–1.

In Table 9–1 net revenue for Hospital A increased $900,000 or 4.50 percent with a 10.0 percent price increase. Net revenue for Hospital B increased only $517,600 or 2.59 percent with the same price increase. This is because only billed-charges payers are affected by price increases. Cost-based payers, bad debts, and charity patients are generally not affected by hospital prices. There are some exceptions to this because of lower-of-cost-or-charges rules, routine service limitations, and other factors associated with cost-reimbursement regulations, but these exceptions are insignificant.

Figure 9–4 Container of Hospital Costs with Billed-Charges Payers at the Economic Spillover Point

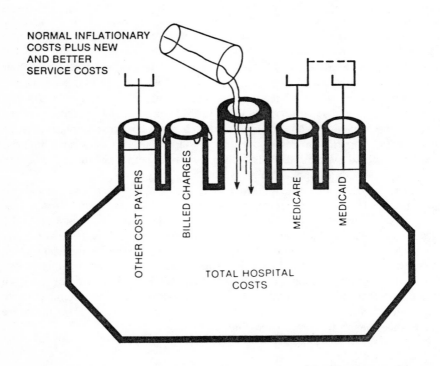

Hospital A will receive billed charges from 45 percent of its patients. In order to effect a 10.00 percent increase in net revenue, it must increase prices an average of 22.22 percent. Hospital B will receive billed charges from only 25 percent of its patients. In order to effect a 10 percent increase in net revenue, it will have to increase prices an average of 40.00 percent. Both hospitals experience the same cost pressures illustrated in Figure 9–4.

There are several strategies that a hospital with a high percentage of cost reimbursement can follow. The first strategy is to reduce the amount of annual cost increases that are added to the container each year. If the hospital reduces the amount spent for new and better services more than other American hospitals, it will soon fall behind. A hospital with outdated equipment and technology will lose the loyalty of its staff physicians. A hospital must therefore be very cautious in determining the amount of reduction in new and better service costs. The hospital can attempt to reduce the amount of normal price increases, but it has only limited control over these increases and the gains will be small.

Table 9–1 Comparative Effect of Hospital Price Increases

Before Price Increase:	Hospital A	Hospital B
Gross billed charges per 100,000 patient days	$20,000,000	$20,000,000
Gross charges to cost payers	10,000,000	10,000,000
Reimbursement from cost payers	−9,000,000	−12,600,000
Contractual allowances	1,000,000	1,400,000
Plus charity and bad debt	+1,000,000	+1,000,000
Total deduction from revenue	2,000,000	2,400,000
Net revenue (Gross charges minus total deductions)	$18,000,000	$17,600,000

After Price Increase:	Hospital A	Hospital B
Gross billed charges per 100,000 patient days	$22,000,000	$22,000,000
Gross charges to cost payers	11,000,000	15,400,000
Reimbursement from cost payers	−9,000,000	−12,600,000
Contractual allowances	2,000,000	2,800,000
Plus charity and bad debt	+1,100,000	+1,100,000
Total deductions from revenue	3,100,000	3,900,000
Net revenue (Gross charges minus total deductions)	$18,900,000	$18,100,000

The hospital can, however, reduce the amount of costs in the container. One way is to become more efficient. But there is a limit to the amount of excess cost, duplication, and other inefficiencies that can be found in any institution. The only other way to make a significant cost reduction in the container is to reverse or take away costs for new and better services that were added in the past. This reduces patient acuity or, in other words, reverses the overall gains made by the hospital in medical technology. Reductions in patient service cannot continue over a long period of time.

As cost reimbursement grows, it will continue to be critical that hospitals maximize the amount they receive from cost reports. In many industries, the difference between bankruptcy, getting by with the least amount of discredit, and success is in the quality of the tax returns. In hospitals, the difference between bankruptcy, getting by with the least amount of discredit, and success is in the quality of the cost reports.

DEFINITION OF COSTS: THE MEDICARE REIMBURSEMENT SYSTEM

Hospitals are reimbursed on the basis of costs by Medicare, Medicaid, and others. The difficulty lies in the definition of costs. Hospitals have a definition of costs in their annual reports. Generally, the annual reports are accompanied by a statement from an independent accounting firm stating that the costs as reported are defined by cost-report principles and are calculated on the basis of generally accepted accounting principles.

Medicare cost reports are universal throughout the United States and are generally the starting point for other cost reports. Other cost systems are either modeled after the Medicare cost-reimbursement system or have many principles in common with those used in Medicare. The Medicare reimbursement system is outlined in Table 9–2. We will examine each of the components of this system to illustrate how cost is defined.

Total Costs

The starting point for total hospital costs is the income statement for the reporting period. Several inputed or allocated costs can be added to this. The first additions that must be considered are related to donations. The hospital is allowed to depreciate donated assets based upon the market value of those assets at the time of donation. Almost every hospital has some assets donated by volunteers, a physician, the community, a business, or by others. Often a hospital will receive substantial aggregated donations from a fund drive. Depreciation from donated assets can be significant.

Hospitals can also add the market value of services performed by certain nonpaid workers. Such workers must work more than 20 hours per week and be in positions that would normally be held by paid personnel.

Table 9–2 The Medicare Cost-Reimbursement System

Total costs	$ XXXXX
Less defined-away cost	XX
Allowable cost	XXXXX
Less offsets and adjustments	XX
Costs to be apportioned	XXXXX
Less apportioned-away costs	XX
Recognized patient costs	XXXXX
Less nonprogram costs	XXX
Allowable costs	XXXXX
Less limits and ceilings	XX
Recognized program costs	XXXX
Plus return on equity	XX
Reimbursable costs	XXXX
Less inflation shrinkage	XX
True reimbursement	$ XXXX

Many hospitals can also add an allocation of corporate overhead. This is used by both chain organizations to distribute corporate costs and by some religious organizations to distribute applicable costs of the motherhouse. Although Blue Cross has the elements of a chain organization task force, techniques used to allocate corporate overhead are not universally defined.

The hospital can also add costs related to the Medicare loss on disposal of assets. This is the difference between the value of assets at the time they are disposed of and the book value shown on the hospital's books. There can also be a Medicare gain on disposal of assets; this must be reported as income by the hospital.

Defined-Away Costs

Once the hospital has determined total costs, it must identify those expenses that by definition are not considered. The regulations define away more costs each year. Some examples of expenses that were considered costs in the past but are not now so considered include allowance in lieu of specific recognition of other costs, accelerated depreciation, and current financing. Allowance in lieu of specific recognition of other costs used to be 2.0 percent for nonprofit hospitals and 1.5 percent for profit hospitals. This was calculated as a percentage of Medicare reimbursement and was intended to pay for the additional administrative expense imposed by Medicare. Accelerated depreciation was allowed to reflect inflation as well as the rapid advances in medical technology. Current financing was a pool of money given to hospitals in order to compensate them for the cost of holding Medicare accounts receivable.

Although bad debts and charity are a cost applicable to all hospitals, these expenses are not recognized for Medicare reimbursement. Medicare bad debts resulting from patient coinsurance and deductibles are an exception to this rule. Medicare bad debts are reimbursable dollar for dollar and are not subject to any apportionment or allocation that may decrease this amount. Some hospitals have classified collection fees as a reduction of bad debts. This should be reclassified to an administrative expense account because collection fees are recognized as an allowable administrative expense. A similar expense is the cost of credit card premiums. This should be called an expense rather than a reduction of revenue. Many Medicare intermediaries do not allow credit-card costs for Medicare, but these may be an allowable cost for another required cost report.

There are many examples of expenses that can be disallowed if treated one way on the hospital's general ledger but will be an allowable expense if handled properly. Some examples are blood administration costs, depreciation and operating cost on nonapproved capital assets, costs of services not considered reasonable and necessary, and the cost of a private room that is considered medically necessary. For example, charges for blood are normally disallowed, but charges for blood administration are allowed.

Depreciation and operating costs on capital assets that exceed $150,000 are allowed only if the hospital has filed a certificate of need and the project was approved by the health planning agency or its successors. Often an expenditure that exceeds this limit can be successfully segregated into several projects, none of which exceed $150,000. If the project cannot be segregated, the hospital should consider professional assistance in completing the certificate-of-need application. Many certificate-of-need applications have been denied because the hospital did an inadequate job of completing the required sections.

To minimize the costs of services not considered reasonable and necessary, the hospital must monitor patient stays by diagnosis and perform medical audits. If a Medicare patient occupies a private room and it is not considered medically necessary, the hospital can bill the patient for the room differential. If the stay is considered medically necessary, the charges for the room differential must be billed to Medicare. Because routine care is reimbursed by Medicare on a per-diem basis rather than on the basis of a ratio of costs to charges, the medically necessary private room does not add to reimbursement. By developing a good rapport with the medical staff, administration can reduce reimbursement losses from these situations.

In the Table 9–2 example, allowable cost is computed by subtracting defined-away cost from total cost.

Offsets and Adjustments

The hospital is required to reduce expenses by many offsets. These include purchase discounts, vending machine rebates, cafeteria income, tuition fees, silver recovery, income from investments except funded depreciation investments, donor gifts designated to support specific operating costs, some payments made to hospital-based physicians, income from television rentals, and other adjustments. Because these miscellaneous income items and savings must be offset against expenses, the hospital does not enjoy the full benefits. For example, if 50 percent of a hospital's patients are Medicare and Medicaid patients, at least 50 percent of the purchase discounts taken will reduce reimbursement. The hospital will benefit only from the purchase discounts that do not reduce reimbursement.

For some of these offsets, the hospital can reduce expenses either by the amount of cash received or by the amount of cost the hospital incurred. In other words, the hospital can make a profit on television rentals, patient telephones, vending machine rebates, and other items if the hospital can identify this profit. Many hospitals offset cash received rather than attempt to identify costs, even though identifying costs generally results in a significantly smaller offset to expenses. It should be cautioned that once an adjustment to expense has been made on the basis of cost, the hospital may not, in the future, use revenue as the basis for that adjustment.

Since income from funded depreciation is not offset on the cost reports if the hospital has investment income every year but does not fund depreciation, it should consider the possibility of starting a funded-depreciation reserve. Restricted gifts should be discouraged if possible since this may reduce cost reimbursement. The hospital can explain Medicare reimbursement to the prospective donor, make either a formal or an implied promise to satisfy the wishes of the donor, and persuade the donor to make an unrestricted donation. As much as possible of the remuneration paid to hospital-based physicians should be allo- *now changed.* cated to administration and teaching rather than direct patient care.

The above represents a few of the techniques that can be used to reduce offsets and adjustments to allowable costs. The hospital should critically examine each offset on an annual basis to identify ways in which these can be reduced.

After substracting offsets and adjustments from allowable costs, the hospital arrives at costs to be apportioned and is ready to begin the step-down process. The step-down process allocates nonrevenue-producing cost centers to the revenue-producing cost centers as overhead.

Apportioned-Away Costs

Apportioned-away costs are the area where reimbursement planning has the greatest potential for gain. The first step in maximizing the amount of costs that will be apportioned to cost reports is to develop a departmental ranking schedule. This is identical to the schedule used in pricing strategy except that here the departments are listed in reverse order. The expense-ranking schedule also includes nonallowable cost centers. Examples of expenses that are not allowable include costs of patient telephones, costs of other personal comfort items, gift shop costs, many family-practice residency costs, and the costs of professional office buildings. The hospital should list all nonallowable cost centers before beginning the apportionment process.

In determining the statistical basis for appointment, those areas that will result in the greatest reimbursement should be favored. As mentioned earlier in connection with pricing strategy, the hospital must not fraudulently weight the statistics. The hospital must always protect its credibility. However. there will be numerous areas in which the hospital can legitimately increase reimbursement through careful planning.

In our example, substracting apportioned-away costs from costs to be apportioned gives recognized patient costs.

Nonprogram Costs

At this point, the Medicare cost report separates out the expenses recognized as patient costs by applying a ratio of charges to charges against costs. In addition to the pricing strategy exercises outlined in the previous chapter, the hospital can charge many expenses in a manner that maximizes the amount received from third party payers.

Reimbursement auditors tend to scrutinize those expense classifications that have been budgeted and charged to a department in the general ledger less than those expenses that have been reclassified on the cost report. For this reason, the hospital should plan reimbursement in the budget process. The general ledger should classify expenses in a manner that will eliminate as many reclassification entries as possible. A reclassification entry is an adjustment on the cost report that moves an expense from one cost center to another. The hospital must support any reclassification entry it makes. By the same logic, if the intermediary makes a reclassification entry that will reduce reimbursement, this reclassification must be supported by the auditor. It is easier and also safer to have expense reclassifications recorded on the general ledger through the hospital's normal accounting process.

The most beneficial placement of expenses depends upon the particular hospital, its departmental ranking schedule, and the reimbursement ceilings imposed by the government. The following examples indicate some reclassifications to consider. It is not, however, a complete list of possible reclassifications.

Social Security, workmen's compensation, unemployment compensation, and other benefits and taxes can either be charged directly to the departments based on actual expenses by department or they can be apportioned. Although the differences by department will be small, they are often significant in total. Emergency room and clinic costs should be analyzed to determine whether some of these expenses can be reclassified as administrative and general. Orderlies and other transportation costs make inpatient ancillary tests more expensive to perform than outpatient tests where the patient is normally ambulatory and walks to the department. Inpatient transportation costs can be charged or expensed separately if they are broken out separately. Some hospitals reclassify the waiting room in the emergency area to administrative and general, combine obstetrical and surgical recovery rooms to reduce delivery expense, reclassify salaries of intravenous teams from nursing to pharmacy, and reclassify salaries for drawing blood samples from nursing to laboratory. Often, anesthetics are purchased through the pharmacy and charged to pharmacy expense rather than to anesthesiology or surgery. The hospital can evaluate whether radiology films or special central supply items used in surgery should be charged to radiology and central supply or to surgery and delivery. The potential for additional reimbursement through careful reclassifications is substantial.

In the Table 9–2 example, substracting nonprogram costs from allowable patient cost produces a tentative reimbursable amount.

Limits and Ceilings

There are several limits and ceilings that can reduce reimbursement below otherwise allowable costs. These are the lower of costs or charges, routine per-diem cost limitations, maximum charges established for many pharmacy items, and expenses that the intermediary determines to be imprudent. At the time of this writing, other limits on hospital costs were being considered by state and federal lawmakers.

The hospital can follow two approaches to reduce the amount of expenses disallowed. The first is to shift costs from one area to another. For example, the operating room is often cleaned by personnel who could be assigned to nursing. As a result of such a shift, there would be less housekeeping cost to allocate to other areas. Similarly, dietary costs can be studied to determine where patient nourishments are charged.

The second approach is to request exceptions or search for pass-throughs. Requests for exceptions are considered on a case-by-case basis. Pass-throughs have been routinely granted for high intern and resident expense per day, for school-of-nursing costs per day, and for malpractice insurance premiums.

Return on Equity

For-profit hospitals receive a return on equity in addition to the amount otherwise claimed for Medicare reimbursement. Nonprofit hospitals do not receive a return on equity. The return on equity is based upon the amount of money invested in fixed assets plus the amount of net working capital. This amount is multiplied by the average interest paid for the past year on government securities.

Because of the return on equity, for-profit hospitals have several accounting policies that differ from those adopted by nonprofit hospitals. The first difference relates to fixed assets. Capitalizing fixed assets is not an advantage for nonprofit hospitals. It would be advantageous if they could expense everything in the year acquired and take this expense on the current-year cost reports. By comparison, a for-profit hospital receives both a return on equity every year that the assets are on the accounting records and an investment credit on its federal income tax. This investment credit is currently ten percent of the cost. The most beneficial asset policy for a nonprofit hospital is to expense as many purchases, remodeling, and repairs as possible. The only exception to this rule is donated assets. A for-profit hospital is allowed to take the cost on market value of donated assets on the cost report as depreciation. The most beneficial asset policy for a for-profit hospital is to capitalize as many purchases, remodeling, and repairs as possible.

Return on equity is calculated on net working capital as well as on fixed assets. Net working capital is the difference between current assets and current liabilities. For-profit hospitals have several financial policies intended either to increase current assets or to decrease current liabilities. For example, current assets can be increased by valuing inventories as high as possible. One way to accomplish this is to inventory supplies located at the nursing stations, include an amount for used linen in the linen inventory, and establish supply inventories in large ancillary departments. Nonprofit hospitals generally expense these inventories. A for-profit hospital will generally have more long-term debt and less short-term debt on the balance sheet than a comparable nonprofit hospital. The reason for this is to increase net working capital. These examples illustrate only a few of the differences between the accounting policies of nonprofit hospitals and those of for-profit hospitals that are intended to increase net working capital. Individually, most of the benefits gained from these different policies are small. In the aggregate, however, the benefits are significant.

Inflation Shrinkage

Because Medicare and other cost reports are based upon the hospital's annual financial statements, final determination of the amount of reimbursement cannot start until several months after the end of the fiscal year. Once the cost report is filed, the intermediary must perform a desk audit, schedule and perform a field audit, and determine proposed audit adjustments. After the proposed audit adjustments are received by the hospital, the controller must evaluate the propriety as well as the effect of the adjustments. The entire process normally takes more than a year and may take several years. During this period of time, the intermediary attempts to withhold funds so that a refund will be due to the hospital at final settlement. No interest is paid on these funds. In the aggregate, they can represent an important source of interest-free borrowings by the federal government. In addition, by repaying the hospital several years after the end of the relevant fiscal year, the government is paying with cheaper money. This is because inflation devalues or makes money cheaper each year.

The hospital should strive to keep this inflation shrinkage to a minimum. One way to do this is by negotiating a high interim rate. The interim rate is the percentage of billed charges that the hospital receives for patient care throughout the year. For example, if the intermediary calculations determine that the hospital's reimbursable cost is approximately 90 percent of its billed charges, the interim rate will be 90 percent. For every $100 in billed charges, the hospital will receive $90. With careful budgeting, the hospital can negotiate a relatively high interim rate.

The hospital can also reduce inflation shrinkage by shortening the cost report audit and appeals process. This is accomplished by preparing accurate, well-documented cost reports and by cooperating as much as possible in the field audit. Discussions with the intermediary concerning proposed adjustments to the cost reports should be timely as well as carefully planned. If the hospital decides to appeal an issue on the cost report, the appeal should be well-documented and professionally presented. Often, by hiring outside assistance, the time it takes to settle an appeal can be shortened and the outcome can be made more favorable to the hospital. There are many attorneys, certified public accounting firms, and consulting firms that specialize in health care.

In the Table 9–2 example, subtracting inflation shrinkage from reimbursable costs gives the true reimbursement that the hospital receives from Medicare program patients.

As noted earlier, Medicaid, many Blue Cross cost contracts, and other cost-based reimbursements are determined in the same manner as Medicare. The Medicare reimbursement system outlined in Table 9–2 determines between 50 and 80 percent of the funds received by American hospitals.

THE COST REPORT PROCESS

In the previous section, it was shown that reimbursement alternatives are most flexible during the hospital cost-reporting year. After the year has ended, it is too late to attempt many of the reporting techniques. In this section, we will examine the Medicare cost report process.

The cost report is normally filed by the hospital based on its accounting year. The Medicare report is due on or before the last day of the third month following the close of the hospital's fiscal year. The intermediary or Social Security agency may grant a one-month extension, but it is not obligated to do so. Most hospitals have selected an intermediary, and reports are filed with this agency. Some hospitals have elected to deal directly with the Social Security agency and file their reports directly with that agency. The appropriate agency must perform an audit within three years of the due date or filing date. After this audit, proposed adjustments are explained to the hospital, and the hospital is given time to evaluate these adjustments. Then the agency schedules an exit conference to discuss the report as adjusted.

If the hospital does not agree with the proposed adjustments and informal discussions with the auditors cannot settle the disagreement, the hospital must wait for an official notice called the Notice of Program Reimbursement. After receiving this notice, the hospital has 180 days to request a hearing.

THE AUDIT PROCESS

Through careful planning, the hospital can minimize adverse adjustments. This section explains the audit process and discusses several techniques that can be used.

Point of View

It is important to keep in mind that throughout the audit process the hospital is in an adversary position with the intermediary. This does not mean that the controller and the director of auditing should not be friendly. It does mean that the controller should remember that, during the audit process, the objectives of the hospital are directly opposed to the objectives of the intermediary or Social Security agency.

To help illustrate this, assume you are negotiating to purchase a new house. You will be friendly and courteous to the seller. However, you will be careful in answering any of the seller's questions, and the seller will also answer your questions carefully. The seller will confirm your answers, and you will probably hire an attorney to protect your interests. If deemed necessary, you may hire an engineer, order a report on the seller's background, and talk to several people in the neighborhood. In an audit of the hospital's cost report, the intermediary and the hospital learn as much as they can about each other, are very careful about the answers they give to each other's questions, and hire outside consultants to assist whenever necessary. In purchasing a house, a person is cautiously friendly with the seller but realizes that the interest of the seller is opposed to the interest of the buyer. In the audit of a cost report, the controller should be friendly and cooperative with the auditors but realize that the interest of the intermediary is opposed to the interest of the hospital.

Preaudit Preparation

Throughout the year, the controller can prepare for the audit by teaching business-office employees, department heads, and administration personnel the basic reimbursement principles. Personnel throughout the hospital are affected by cost reimbursement; their daily decisions will determine the amount of reimbursement the hospital will receive. The hospital can maximize reimbursement during the audit by having a well-informed team of hospital personnel. Often controllers will explain reimbursement to supervisors in the business office or to department heads and believe they have done their job. It is not enough, however, to explain reimbursement principles. The controller is also responsible for the actions of others. If controllers do not achieve understanding of the audit process, they will have failed. This understanding is especially important in preaudit planning because a misinformed person can inadvertently cost the hospital thousands of dollars in reimbursement.

When the hospital is notified of an upcoming field audit by Medicare or other major third party agency, the controller should schedule a preaudit strategy conference. This conference should include supervisors from accounting, payroll, credit, billing, accounts payable, cashiering, and data processing. In smaller hospitals, one person may supervise more than one of the functions. This strategy meeting should be scheduled to take place the week before the field audit. At this meeting, the supervisors should be instructed on how to respond to the auditor's questions. Weak points as well as strong points in the cost report can be discussed. There will be some areas in which the controller will want the auditors to spend a great deal of time and other areas in which the controller does not want the auditors to spend time. These should be discussed and strategies should be formulated to accomplish the desired results. If known, the personalities of the auditors can be discussed. The purpose of the preaudit strategy conference is to prepare for the audit in order to be able to control the direction and, therefore, the outcome as much as possible.

The Field Audit

The field audit forms the basis for the proposed-adjustments and appeal process. There are several basic rules that the hospital can follow to control this portion of the cost report process.

Third party auditors should not be allowed to request information from any hospital employee except the supervisors from the financial area who were in attendance at the planning conference. Nonroutine questions should be answered only by the controller or other person thoroughly familiar with Medicare principles. The auditors should not walk around the hospital without an escort from the financial area. If the auditors need photocopies, the copies should be prepared by a clerk who should make a list of all information given to the auditors.

Throughout the field audit, the controller should schedule regular meetings with the audit supervisor. The progress of the audit as well as any proposed audit adjustments should be discussed. If the field audit is to last several weeks, the controller should also meet with the financial area supervisors to discuss the progress of the audit. At the completion of the audit, the controller and supervisors should hold a postaudit planning conference.

The importance of planning and controlling the field audit cannot be overemphasized. It is during this period that support is gathered for any appeals that the hospital may ultimately make on proposed adjustments.

Proposed Adjustments

Proposed audit adjustments do not represent law or Medicare regulations. When they are first presented to the hospital, audit adjustments represent the opinions of the auditors and should be reviewed as opinions. Each year the chief financial officer should carefully review the proposed adjustments to determine their effect on reimbursement. They should be examined to determine whether the auditor acted on incomplete or inaccurate information. If the information was correct, the hospital should determine whether it agrees with the adjustment. Favorable audit adjustments are sometimes contested by the hospital.

If the adjustment will have an unfavorable effect upon reimbursement, the chief financial officer should automatically oppose the adjustment and attempt to develop a case to oppose it. Many hospitals routinely accept adverse audit adjustments when they are supported by a reference to an intermediary letter, a code section, or a court decision. This posture is wrong because it inhibits creative thinking. By aggressively researching support to oppose each adverse audit adjustment, the controller will often find contraregulations, arguments to negate the conclusions in intermediary letters, and other court decisions that support the hospital's viewpoint. The hospital should attempt to develop a case to oppose audit adjustments proposed in prior years as well as those proposed for the first time. Often, only after several years will a hospital be able to develop arguments that can be used to negate successfully an adverse adjustment.

If the hospital decides to appeal a proposed audit adjustment beyond the exit conference, the intermediary will perform additional research to support its position and often will seek legal advice. In order to succeed, the hospital must also perform additional research to support its position. Often the side that performs the most creative research wins. If significant dollars are involved, the hospital should retain outside professional help. Many law firms, certified public accountants, and consulting firms have health-care reimbursement specialists. These specialists can assist in formulating strategy and in negotiating as well as in constructing the appeal.

SUMMARY

Each year American hospitals experience two different kinds of cost increases. Inflation has historically accounted for about two-thirds of the annual increases. These inflation increases are experienced by all industries. Approximately one-third of the average cost increase in hospitals each year can be attributed to new and better services. New and better services include new tests and procedures as well as increases in the number of tests performed per patient day.

Cost-based payers can effectively transfer part of the costs attributable to their patients or to another class of patient by not allowing all of the cost increases to flow through the cost reports. This increases the cost to billed-charges patients. As long as a third party payer does not reimburse the hospital on billed charges, there is a chance that payer will not absorb all of the costs applicable to its patients.

Hospital price increases generally only affect that class of patients who pay billed charges. Price increases do not affect cost-based payers, charity, or bad-debt patients.

Cost payers do not reimburse based on the definition of costs defined by generally accepted accounting principles. They reimburse costs as defined in a contract, a law, or a regulation. For Medicare and Medicaid reimbursement, the following are substracted from total costs to arrive at true reimbursement: defined-away costs; offsets and adjustments; apportioned-away costs; nonprogram costs; limits and ceilings, and inflation shrinkage costs. There are specific strategies and techniques that a hospital should follow to minimize the amount of money lost in the cost report process.

After its fiscal year end, the hospital prepares cost reports with an intermediary. The intermediary audits the cost report and prepares a list of proposed audit adjustments. At this point, the hospital and the intermediary are in adversary positions. The objectives of the hospital throughout the audit process are directly opposed to the objectives of the auditors. The hospital should carefully plan for the audit in order to maintain control of the information given to auditors.

Proposed audit adjustments should be viewed as merely the opinions of the auditors. Carefully coordinated examination of each proposed audit adjustment will often reveal new ways to appeal or negotiate the adjustments. It is often helpful to obtain outside professional assistance. Many law firms, certified public accountants, and consulting firms have health-care reimbursement specialists.

DISCUSSION QUESTIONS

1. Explain normal hospital cost increases. Contrast these increases with those associated with new and better services.
2. How can cost-based payers shift a portion of their proportionate share of the costs of providing hospital services to the billed charges payers?
3. When determining price increases, why does a hospital with a large percentage of billed-charges patients have a decided advantage over a hospital with a large percentage of cost-based patients?
4. List and discuss four of the reductions from total costs that are made during the Medicare cost report process.
5. List several strategies the hospital can adopt to minimize reductions from total costs.
6. Define an effective point of view that the hospital can adopt toward the intermediary or the Social Security agency during the audit and final settlement of the Medicare cost report.
7. List some preaudit preparations that the hospital can adopt to assist in controlling the field audit.
8. How should a hospital evaluate proposed audit adjustments?

Chapter 10

Purchasing and Accounts Payable

In this chapter we examine financial controls over purchasing and accounts payable. To understand the importance of these controls, assume a hospital has a net gain on gross revenue of five percent. In this case, a diversion of $1,000 in funds is equal to $20,000 in lost charges. In other words, a saving of $1,000 through purchasing controls has the same impact as $20,000 in new program revenue. Purchasing and accounts payable controls affect the bottom line of the income statement dollar for dollar.

PURCHASING

Every function that the purchasing department performs is for other departments. If purchasing can improve management practices throughout the hospital, the end result will be savings to all departments. In this section, we will look at ways in which this can be accomplished.

Purchasing Function

Control starts when goods or services are ordered and continues through the receipt and use of the goods or services. The diagram in Figure 10–1 will be used to describe the process as well as to illustrate what check points contribute to internal control.

As shown on the Figure 10–1 flow chart, the purchasing function begins with a department sending a purchase requisition to purchasing. The purchasing department selects a vendor and prepares a multipart purchase order. One copy of the purchase order is returned to the requesting department to indicate that the goods or services have been ordered. A copy of the purchase order is sent to accounts payable and another to the vendor. A copy of the purchase order is also sent to receiving to match against the shipment when it is delivered. The

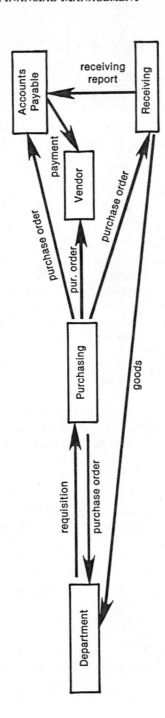

Figure 10–1 Procurement Flow Chart

vendor fills the order and sends an invoice to accounts payable. When accounts payable has a proper receiving report, invoice, and purchase order, payment is sent to the vendor. The goods received are sent to the department that originated the request. If the purchase order was for services, there may not be a receiving report; in this case, the vendor performs the service directly for the requesting department.

In implementing the purchasing function, it is assumed that the purchasing department makes decisions; it is not simply an order-placing agency. It is also assumed that the purchasing department is regarded by department heads as an information center for all types of goods or services. An effective centralized purchasing system will save the hospital thousands of dollars annually.

The first responsibility of those directing the purchasing function is to implement an inventory control system. This responsibility is shared with user departments, but purchasing must take the lead in developing economic order quantities, safety stocks, and vendor lead times. However, not all items should be controlled. Hospitals use an extraordinary variety of supply items. The unit costs of many of these items are too small to justify the adoption of sophisticated control methods. It is the responsibility of purchasing to develop an acquired or an intuitive time-value ratio for hospital supply items. Is the dollar value of this item large enough to justify inventory control? Is the potential for savings significant, or are the prices of these items relatively inflexible? If the potential for gain is not significant, the supply item is not worth the time needed to control it.

The specification of brand name versus generic name for an item is another part of the purchasing function. Whenever possible, unless the difference in quality is unacceptable, items should be ordered by generic name rather than brand name. To make this determination, the hospital will have a product evaluation committee. This committee should be chaired by the purchasing director, and at least one member should be a physician who has excellent rapport with the medical staff. The product evaluation committee should be user oriented but at the same time be aware of the fact that many hospital employees have the incorrect notion that the hospital should always purchase the highest quality possible. Often items of lower quality, and therefore lower price, can be substituted with no effect on patient care. The hospital does not need the highest quality stationary, office supplies, linen, disposables, and other such items. Many lab tests can be performed with several different kinds of high grade chemicals with no decrease in clinical quality. Often more expensive diagnostic equipment adds very little to the clinical quality of the test results. The mystique that everything in a hospital must be of the highest quality available simply is not true.

Because purchasing performs all of its functions for the benefit of another department, it is important that the personnel in purchasing be user oriented.

This is accomplished in many ways. Purchase requests should always be executed in a timely manner to avoid out-of-stock situations as well as to gain enough confidence to prevent departments from overstocking. Whenever possible, models and demonstrators should be requested on a trial basis before purchase. This is especially true for large equipment items. This allows the department to evaluate the product before purchasing and at the same time delays the outlay of cash. Even if the hospital is sure that it will purchase a piece of equipment and has agreed upon a firm price, many purchasing agents will negotiate a trial period and effectively delay payment for two months or more. Another way in which purchasing can assist other departments is by maintaining a vendor performance file. This file will enable purchasing to answer questions and to give advice to department heads about vendor performance, flexibility, quality and promptness of service, and other matters.

A good purchasing department provides other departments with the tools needed to budget accurately. Purchasing can also reduce budget variances and assist in explaining the reasons for budget variances throughout the fiscal year.

Requisitions

As noted, a requisition originates from the user department. The first control over requisitions is an approved list of designated persons who are authorized to initiate a purchase request. This departmental list normally includes the department head and one or more other persons within the department. By formalizing this list into an approved policy, the hospital gains an important aspect of internal control as well as a saving in time and questions from both purchasing and user departments.

The hospital should also have an approved and functioning policy on approvals for capital equipment requisitions. The purchase of a capital item is a long-range decision, and requisitions for such items generally need a higher approval than those for supplies.

Requisitions are also controlled by dollar amount. Over a set dollar limit, the purchase requisition must be signed by a department head. Over a higher set limit, the purchase requisition must be approved by administration. Generally the hospital will have one set of approval levels for capital items and another for noncapital items.

Vendor salespersons on the nursing floors and in the hospital departments demand a good deal of the time of hospital personnel. Much of this time is necessary in order for the hospital to remain technologically competitive. Much of this time is not necessary, however, and is an imposition upon those department managers who do not know how to say no. To control this, all salespersons should be required to sign in and out with purchasing. The purchasing director can turn away those who department managers do not want to see or can reschedule a call for a time when the department head is less busy.

Departments should be instructed that under no circumstances should they tell a salesperson that they will purchase a product. All purchasing should be done by the purchasing department. This is important because once salespeople know that their product is the only acceptable brand, all price negotiating leverage has been lost. Professional purchasing agents can talk about alternative products and negotiate lower prices even though they are talking to the vendor who supplies the only acceptable product at the time. Professional price negotiating can produce significant cost savings for the hospital.

There are three exceptions to centralized purchasing in most hospitals. These are in pharmacy, dietary, and maintenance. Drugs are usually purchased by a registered pharmacist. Many drugs cannot legally be purchased by a nonpharmacist. Dietary menu items are purchased by the person who plans the menu. In that way, the hospital can alter menus to take advantage of special price reductions. Maintenance often needs a part or a service call on very short notice. The routine purchasing process takes too much time in these instances. Maintenance personnel must always have the ability to make purchases quickly when they are performing emergency repairs.

However, pharmacy, dietary, and maintenance departments should be allowed to purchase directly pharmacy drugs, dietary menu items, and maintenance repair items only when it is expedient or less expensive to do so. All other purchases made by these departments should be processed by a centralized purchasing department.

Control over purchases made directly by other departments is exercised in two ways. The first is through purchase orders. Purchasing assigns all purchase order numbers and gives other departments purchase order numbers that they may use. Copies of completed purchase orders are sent by other departments to purchasing for review after the purchase. The second control exerted directly on other departments is through an administrative policy giving the purchasing director authority to audit and report on vendor selection, buying habits, and pricing. This authority is not given in all hospitals, and its absence results in higher prices. When allowed to audit the procurement practices of pharmacy, dietary, and maintenance, the purchasing director acts as a management consultant and source of information that can improve the business practices of these departments.

Common and recurring purchase requests from hospital departments can be effectively organized on a standard order form on which the department manager can check those items needed. All other purchase requisitions should be on a standard hospital form used by all departments. Telephone requests to purchasing should be followed by a completed purchase requisition. Once received, the purchasing department should review all requisitions before placing an order. This review should include a determination of reasonableness for the item ordered. A nursing station should not have a large order for envelopes, and the business office should not have a large order for dressings or other medical supplies. The review should also question excessive quantities of items that the hospital may not be able to use. If the purchase requisition is proper, a purchase order is prepared.

Purchase Orders

A purchase order should be completed for all items, including services, ordered through the purchasing department. Items ordered over the telephone should be followed up with a purchase order. This document should show a complete description of the items ordered, the prices with applicable discounts noted, and the terms. The purchase orders should be sequentially numbered and all numbers accounted for, including voided numbers.

In completing a purchase order, the purchasing agent must first decide exactly what will be ordered. Can the item be ordered from a catalog, or will the hospital request competitive bids? Should the order be for a brand name or a generic name? Can a similar item be substituted that will meet the needs of several departments?

Many hospitals maintain an approved vendor list, and purchases can be processed only through a vendor on this list. Whether or not there is a formal list, the hospital should only buy from reputable vendors.

There are several important business practices to keep in mind if the purchase order is to be sent out for competitive bids. One is to consider all provisions of the bid when making comparisons. This includes freight, set up, lead time, terms, discounts, and services. Often the vendor submitting the lowest bid is not offering the lowest price after considering all factors of the purchase. Another practice is to open negotiations after competitive bids have been examined. For example, the purchasing agent can call the second lowest vendor and negotiate a lower price using the low bid as leverage. Then the former low-bid vendor can be called. This technique cannot be used every time because it will tempt vendors to bid high in quotations to the hospital. However, for an occasional significant purchase, working the price of a bid down can result in substantial savings to the hospital.

Most items are purchased from a catalog rather than in a bidding process. This can be a supplier's catalog or a catalog of group-purchasing prices negotiated by a hospital association, central office, or other entity. The hospital should have an adequate library of catalogs and current price lists for all items. A lack of a good catalog library indicates the purchasing department is not performing enough exploratory work prior to placing orders. Old price catalogs should be purged regularly to avoid costly purchasing. If a frequently used vendor regularly distributes a new catalog, such as annually or semiannually, the expected date of the new catalog should be carefully monitored. If the hospital can predict the date price increases will go into effect, it may be beneficial to stockpile items by placing a large order just prior to the effective date of the price increase. This will be advantageous, however, only if the amount of the price increase is great enough to offset the temporary loss of working capital.

Sometimes it is not expedient to solicit formal bids when an item is not included in one of the vendor or hospital association catalogs. This is often the case when purchasing a service. In such cases, the purchasing agent should obtain quotations from several vendors. These quotations should be well-documented and not discarded after the purchase is made. The documented quotations become the audit support for the purchase. Medicare auditors can disallow the expenses of a purchase if the hospital cannot prove it was prudent. Outside auditors often comment negatively if documentation for all purchases is not available. In addition, the purchasing agent can use the telephone quotation file when researching vendors to place future orders.

In choosing vendors and negotiating terms for items, the hospital should attempt to have two or more sources for critical supplies. There are two major advantages to be gained by having alternate sources. First, the hospital reduces the chance of being cut off by a strike, by low vendor inventory, or by some other nonpredictable reason. Second, having an alternate source serves as a channel to keep price negotiations open with the primary supplier. If an extraordinary price increase is imposed, the hospital can quickly change to the alternate supplier.

Purchasing must know when to place an order. This requires knowing both the vendors and the department heads. If purchasing does not keep the paperwork smooth and timely, departments will go outside the purchasing organization and purchase directly. Even with approved hospital policies and procedures, the practice of direct department purchasing is very difficult to control. If purchasing places all orders when received, the hospital may have excessive inventories of some supplies, because some departments have a tendency to overorder while others may send a completed purchase requisition to purchasing only when a stockout is imminent. By matching the purchasing tendencies of department heads with the order-filling processes of vendors, the purchasing director can keep inventories down and at the same time avoid an out-of-stock situation for a needed item.

Preprinted purchase orders are used for frequently ordered items. These are often different in format and have a unique sequence of numbers that is different from that used on the standard purchase orders. This is because they are custom-made for a particular vendor or a particular item. It is important to remember that the multicopy needs of preprinted purchase orders are the same as that of standard forms. Copies are sent to the vendor, accounts payable, originating hospital department, and receiving, and one copy is retained in purchasing files.

Purchasing Controls

In previous sections, we examined many operating procedures that also serve as purchasing controls. Because these procedures serve more than one purpose, they will be reexamined here in relation to purchasing controls.

It is important that the purchasing department initiate a purchase order on all procurements. These include services, telephone orders, and purchases by other departments. For selective purchasing done by pharmacy, dietary, and maintenance, the purchasing department should issue and control the purchase order numbers. One way is to issue these departments small blocks of purchase order numbers in sequence and to account for all numbers issued, including those for voided purchase orders. Control is then completed by enforcing a policy that prohibits accounts payable from issuing a check for any nonsalary item unless the invoice is accompanied by a purchase order.

The completed purchase order should give a complete description, the price or prices, and the terms of the item or service being purchased. A dollar and percentage price variance should be established. For example, the hospital might define a variance of two percent or one hundred dollars, whichever is lowest. Accounts payable then will not pay any invoice in which the difference between the invoice amount and the purchase order amount is greater than this variance. Invoices that exceed the variance will be sent by accounts payable to purchasing. Purchasing will then either contact the vendor or approve the new price. The important point is that purchasing is controlling the price paid and has a chance to change its price lists if a higher price is approved. By approving price variances on an exception basis, the purchasing department is approving all invoice prices without signing each invoice.

Purchasing should be separated from receiving—functionally, organizationally, and in the flow of paperwork to accounts payable. Purchasing and receiving must work together with other departments in inventory control, but their respective input should be separated. Separation of duties is a major element of internal control over the purchasing function.

Control over vendors is effected in several ways. One way is by establishing an approved vendor list with the required criteria. Another is by enforcing a policy and procedure to control the time as well as the activities of salespeople throughout the hospital. If the hospital has more than one supplier for major supply items, there is an element of control over vendor pricing. Most hospitals also maintain by vendor a year-to-date balance of dollars purchased. This is usually a part of the accounts payable function. Knowing how many dollars worth of orders the hospital has placed with a vendor is also useful information for purchasing to have when negotiating prices and terms of a purchase.

Purchasing should have specific policies and procedures to control vendor backorders, pending-shipment files, partial shipments, and other matters that can cause purchase orders to remain open for an excessive period of time. These policies and procedures should guarantee regular review of the reasons for open-purchase orders. Information gained from these reviews is used to update vendor performance files, to monitor hospital errors, and to guarantee that the system of numerical control of all purchase orders is not being abused.

All of the controls over the purchasing function should be established through an approved policy and procedure. If the hospital does not have an extensive policy and procedure system to definitively spell out these controls, it must rely on memorandums and verbal instructions that tend to become unclear over time.

ACCOUNTS PAYABLE

Accounts payable is the focal point of all nonsalary expenditures. This function processes checks, enforces controls, and performs the final audit of account distribution.

Accounts Payable Function

Accounts payable processes both notes and accounts that are currently payable. These originate from the purchase of goods, equipment, and services and from borrowing. Notes currently payable can be from short-term borrowings, or they may represent the current portion of long-term debt. In presenting current payables on the balance sheet, notes payable are normally classified separately from accounts payable.

The accounts payable function begins when a copy of the completed purchase order is received from the purchasing department. This is filed alphabetically by vendor in an unrecorded-liability or incomplete-payables file. As goods, equipment, and services are received, a copy of the receiving report or other document acknowledging that the hospital has incurred a liability is matched to the purchase order. At that point, the purchase order represents an unrecorded liability. As invoices are received, a search is made in the unrecorded liabilities file for a purchase order and either a receiving report or an appropriate substitute document.

If an invoice contains items that were received but not ordered, the invoice and receiving report are given to purchasing for approval or other disposition. Purchasing must also approve the payment if the billed price exceeds the purchase order price by more than a predetermined limit. If the invoice contains items that were ordered but not received, a debit memo is prepared and attached to the invoice. A debit memo is also prepared for items that were neither ordered nor received.

After matching the purchase order, receiving document, and invoice, the accounts payable clerk audits the invoice for accuracy, checking quantity, price, extensions, and discounts. The general ledger account or accounts that will be charged is verified, and the invoice is set up for payment. This includes recording the liability, determining a date for payment, and, depending upon the hospital's policy, either approving the invoice or sending the invoice to the proper person outside the accounts payable section for approval.

Special procedures are needed to handle payments for which there is no invoice. The hospital should have a check request form that undergoes the same kind of audit and approval as an invoice. The check request form merely substitutes for an invoice. Payments made without an invoice include payments on loans, employee travel advances, reimbursement of petty cash funds, some professional fees in which the hospital calculates the amount owed, certain regular contractual amounts, and other payments.

Timing of Payables

It is the responsibility of accounts payable to record all liabilities and to process checks for payment at the proper time. For accounting reasons, the recording of liabilities must be in the proper period. The processing of payments must be properly timed because of cash considerations.

A good rule to follow is to delay payments until the last possible day. That is the last day on which the hospital can take a purchase discount if one is offered. If no purchase discount is offered, it is the last day on which the hospital can pay the obligation and still be considered current. By delaying payment, the hospital is, in effect, increasing its available cash. If the hospital can delay its disbursements by an average of two days, it has increased available cash by two times the average daily cash outflow. If the hospital can delay its disbursements by an average of three days, it has increased available cash by three times the average daily cash outflow.

It is important for the hospital to take all available cash discounts, even if it is necessary to borrow funds from the bank to do this. The reason for this is that, if a hospital misses a purchase discount, it is in effect paying an excessively high interest rate. To illustrate this, assume that the terms of an invoice are 2/ 10 net 30. This means that the hospital can take a two percent discount if it pays within 10 days and that the net amount is due by the end of the 30th day. In effect, the hospital would be paying two percent interest if it decided to forgo the discount and keep the funds for the additional 20 days. If we assume 360 days in a year, the interest rate can be calculated as follows:

$$\frac{360 \text{ days}}{20 \text{ days}} \times 2 \text{ percent} = 36 \text{ percent}$$

By missing the purchase discount, the hospital paid an effective 36 percent interest rate for the use of the funds for an additional 20 days. Clearly, this is an excessive interest rate and the hospital would have been ahead by borrowing money at bank interest rates to pay within the discount period.

As invoices are processed for payment, the known dollar amount is set up as a liability. In addition, the hospital will have many accrued liabilities. These are obligations for goods or services that were received but either the vendor has not sent an invoice or the due date for payment is sometime in the future. Some examples of nonsalary accrued liabilities are items received but not invoiced, sales tax collections, use taxes if applicable, liabilities under bonus agreements or physician guarantee arrangements, patient deposits, estimated contingent liabilities, estimated real estate, personal property or income taxes if applicable, and patient refunds.

The nonsalary accrued liability that is the most significant is unrecorded accounts payable. These are calculated by examining the unrecorded-liabilities file at the end of each month. A schedule is made of all purchase orders with attached receiving documents. This schedule represents goods and services that have been received but not invoiced. A journal entry is made to record these items. If the amount is not known exactly, an estimate is made. This entry is reversed in the following month because, when the invoice is received and processed for payment, an account will be assigned. If the accrued liability is not reversed, we would be expensing the invoice twice. At the end of the hospital's fiscal year, a more intensive effort is made to identify unrecorded accounts-payable liabilities to guarantee a more accurate cutoff.

Disbursements by Check

Just prior to the payment date, the accounts payable department removes the vendor package from the files to be processed for payment. This package includes the purchase order, receiving document, and invoice. The package indicates the account or accounts to be charged. It shows that extensions, discounts, and prices have been checked and that all applicable approvals for payment have been received. Many hospitals use a rubber stamp on the face of the invoice. Exhibit 10-1 is an example of a stamp used to indicate approval of an invoice. As each step is completed, the employee should initial the appropriate item on the voucher or audit block, thereby fixing responsibility for performance of that step.

Except for small amounts paid out of petty cash, all hospital disbursements should be made by check. The cancelled check serves as an important control document as well as an effective receipt for payments made. As checks are prepared, the invoice, receiving report, purchase order, and all other supporting documents should be cancelled. The check amount is entered by vendor into a ledger that provides a record of year-to-date purchases by vendor. These vendor summarizations are used by purchasing in negotiations with salespeople. The check is prepared by accounts payable in some hospitals and by the accounting department in other hospitals.

Exhibit 10-1 Accounts Payable Approval Stamp

Received
Purchase Order
Prices
Extension/Footings

Discount
    Computed by
    Amount

Distribution   Account(s)
Approved

Vendor checks should always be signed and mailed by a person outside of the accounts payable function. Until they are mailed, the signed checks should be controlled by the signer or by someone not in the earlier chain of events. They should not be returned to accounts payable for mailing. In most hospitals, accounts payable checks are signed with a signature plate or rubber stamp. As they are signed, a log should be kept of check numbers. Since checks are numerically sequenced, the missing numbers on the check-signing log should equal the voided checks. If a check is not signed and not on the voided check list, the omission should be investigated.

Petty Cash

Most hospitals have one or more petty cash accounts to pay for goods and services that are small in amount and for which payment must be made quickly. The most common petty cash funds are in receiving, to pay for small freight bills; in maintenance, for hardware and other small supplies; in central supply, for miscellaneous purchases; and with the hospital cashier, for all petty cash disbursements not made out of other petty cash funds.

All petty cash funds should be reimbursed as necessary at the end of each month. At year end, all petty cash funds should be reimbursed in order to distribute the expenses to the proper accounts. Reimbursement checks should be made out to the custodian of the fund who endorses and cashes the check.

Petty cash funds are established at an imprest amount. All disbursements should be recorded on a petty cash voucher that is signed by the person receiving the cash. The amount of cash plus signed vouchers should always equal the petty cash imprest amount.

Debit Memos

Credits and refunds from vendors represent a significant problem for hospitals because of the diverse variety of supply, service, and equipment items received. These credits and refunds are best controlled by issuing an instant debit memo that claims a credit against the next invoice paid to the vendor. A debit memo is initiated by purchasing and processed by accounts payable as a debit to the vendor's appropriate general ledger account. Hence the name debit memo.

Exhibit 10–2 is an example of a debit memo for Community Hospital. It contains a number that is used for reference and the vendor's name and address. The description section has five subsections: the quantity of items; the unit of measure, which can be each, carton, dozen, pound, or other unit; a description of the item or items; the unit price; and the extended amount. In our example, the hospital can claim a credit for up to three different kinds of items on one debit memo. The remarks section is used to describe the reason for claiming a credit. Some common reasons are a difference in a price as quoted and billed, a shipment that is not complete, a shipment refused, items returned, damaged or spoiled goods, and a hospital's special discount not honored.

The alternative to issuing an instant debit memo is to call or write the vendor to ask for an adjustment on the next invoice. This must then be filed and monitored to determine when the credit is issued. This is very time-consuming and often requires a follow-up action before a credit is actually issued. With a debit memo, the hospital claims the credit and it is up to the vendor to accept or refuse it. Most claims for credit will be honored by the vendor. Those that are not honored should be sent to the purchasing department for further action.

EMPLOYEE BONDING

Need for Bonding

An important responsibility of management is to provide fidelity bonds to cover employees who handle the assets of the hospital. This protects the hospital against loss from purchasing and accounts-payable employees as well as other employees. These include cashiers and personnel in administration, receiving, stores, and other departments. Other advantages of bonding employees are in the psychological deterrent that bonding carries with it and from the investigation

Exhibit 10–2 Debit Memo Form

DEBIT MEMO
Community Hospital   No. _____
Credit Memorandum

Vendor: Name _____

         Address _____

                 _____

Please process a credit to our account for the following items:

Quantity	U/M	Description	Unit Price	Amount

                                    Total Credit $ _____

Remarks:

                    Prepared by:
                    Approved by:

that bonding companies often make of employees in order to keep the risk of loss to a minimum.

The fact that all employees are highly trusted is not a substitute for bonding. It is an established fact that most fraud is committed by trusted employees, because they have the greatest opportunity. It is usually events away from the hospital that trigger the illegal or criminal act. This could be a severe personal financial crisis, like a major illness, or it could be a behavioral problem. In many instances, there is a careful record of the amounts stolen that indicates there was a sincere intent to pay the hospital back when things improved. In other instances, the person is a disgruntled employee who does not feel fairly compensated. Such employees convince themselves that rather than stealing they are merely taking what rightfully belongs to them. In view of these uncontrollable risk factors, fidelity insurance is indispensable to the hospital.

Kinds of Bonds

Fidelity bonds are in reality more like insurance policies than bonds. In general, the coverage protects the hospital against loss of money, securities, equipment, supplies, or other property as a result of a dishonest act by a bonded employee. There are several clauses in a fidelity bond that should be clearly understood. The insuring clause recites the causes of loss covered by the bond. The salvage clause provides the method by which any recovered money or property will be distributed. The discovery clause defines the period in which a loss can be discovered and still be insured. This may be during the life of the bond or within a definite period after termination. The continuous liability clause is used with bonds that supersede cancelled bonds. It makes the new bond cover a loss that happened during the time the previous bond was in force and that would have been covered under that bond had it been discovered within the discovery period.

An individual bond covers the hospital against a dishonest or criminal act of a named employee. The act may be made by the employee acting alone or in collusion with others while the named employee holds any position at any location in the hospital. There is usually a valuable investigation made into the background of the specific employee.

A name-schedule bond covers two or more employees. The name-schedule bond provides the same protection as an individual form but includes the name of two or more employees in a schedule. The amount for which each employee is bonded is included in the schedule. The advantage of the schedule is the ease with which changes can be made in the amounts of coverage and additions, deletions, or substitutions made to the schedule of employees. These are all accomplished by endorsements. Cancellation and rewriting is necessary if individual bonds are used.

The position bond covers employees in certain named positions even though the individuals holding these positions change. No followup is required to keep up with employee turnover because the insurance company is relying upon the judgment of the hospital in selecting employees. The additional cost of this kind of bond should be compared with the cost of processing applicable endorsements on a name-schedule bond. If turnover of employees covered under the bond is relatively infrequent, the hospital should obtain a name-schedule bond rather than a position bond.

A blanket bond covers all officers and employees of the hospital. Insurance may be provided for all employees up to the covered amount of the bond. This is called a blanket-position bond. Another type of blanket bond covers all employees in the aggregate up to the covered amount. This is called a primary commercial blanket bond. The premiums are higher on a blanket-position bond because the bond amount could be paid on every employee for a common loss. Individual investigations are normally not made for either type of blanket bond. The costs are normally not high on a per-capita basis because the hospital is covering positions, such as in housekeeping or maintenance, in which there is less opportunity to commit a significant act of fraud.

Some hospitals rely on their insurance underwriter to select the coverage and the kinds of fidelity bonds they purchase. As a result, they often pay for coverage they do not need and are inadequately covered in positions in which opportunities for fraud are greatest. Using the basic principles outlined in this section as a guide, the hospital's chief financial officer should review fidelity-bond coverage annually to determine the needs of the institution. These needs should be compared to existing coverage with appropriate changes made.

SUMMARY

Every function performed by the purchasing department is for the benefit of other departments. Controls and improved business practices in purchasing therefore improve the entire hospital. The purchasing function starts with a requisition from the user department. A purchase order is prepared, and copies are sent to the requesting department, accounts payable, and receiving as well as to the vendor. The focal point of control in this process is accounts payable.

Purchasing can employ many business practices that will lower costs without sacrificing quality. One technique is to purchase by generic name rather than brand name whenever possible. The acceptance of this practice can be aided by establishing a product-acceptance committee. Another practice is to purchase products that are common and acceptable to several departments.

Purchase requisitions should be accepted only from those on an approved list of designated hospital personnel who have authority to initiate a request. This practice is an important aspect of internal control as well as a time-saving procedure for both purchasing and user departments. Orders should be placed only with vendors who are on the hospital's approved vendor list. This list should be flexible, and additions should be made freely. The purposes of the approved vendor list are to make purchasing more efficient and to ensure that the hospital buys only from reputable vendors.

Purchasing should control all contact with vendors in order to negotiate the lowest cost. Salespeople should register with purchasing before visiting department heads, and all price negotiating should be performed by purchasing.

A purchase order should be completed for all items ordered through the purchasing department. This includes services and orders negotiated over the telephone. The purchase order gives a complete description of the product terms, prices, and discounts if applicable. Preprinted purchase orders are used for frequently ordered items.

All of the controls over purchasing and accounts payable should be established through an approved policy and procedure system. Otherwise controls will be exercised through memorandums and verbal instructions that tend to become unclear over a period of time.

Accounts payable is the focal point of all nonsalary expenditures. This function processes checks, enforces controls, and makes the final determination of the general ledger account to be charged. Checks are not prepared until the hospital has matched a receiving report, purchase order, and invoice. Any discrepancy noted in matching these three documents should be cleared up before the check is prepared. Payment of payables should be delayed until the last possible day. However, discounts should be taken even if the hospital must borrow funds to pay within the discount period. If a hospital misses a purchase discount, it is effectively paying an excessively high interest rate.

The amount of formal internal control procedures used will depend upon the particular hospital. It should be noted that it is a duty and responsibility of management to help all employees keep themselves honest through establishing and maintaining proper internal controls.

Credits and refunds due from vendors are best controlled by issuing an instant debit memo that claims a credit against the next invoice paid to the vendor. A debit memo is initiated by purchasing and processed by accounts payable.

The hospital should review its fidelity bond coverage annually to compare the needs of the institution to existing coverage. There are four major kinds of bonds: individual bond, name-schedule bond, position bond, and blanket bond. Each of these will contain an insuring clause, salvage clause, discovery clause, and continuous liability clause.

DISCUSSION QUESTIONS

1. Why is it important for the purchasing department to take the lead in establishing sound business practices?
2. Give a brief narrative outline of the procurement function.
3. Name some things that should be considered by a good purchasing department before processing a purchase requisition received from a department.
4. What are some purchasing controls that the hospital can initiate?
5. Give a brief narrative outline of the accounts payable function.
6. When should invoices from vendors be processed for payment?

7. How do petty cash funds operate? How are they reimbursed?
8. What is the purpose of fidelity bonds in a hospital whose employees are all loyal and trusted?
9. Explain the difference between a primary commercial blanket bond and a blanket-position bond.

Chapter 11

Receiving and Inventory Management

In this chapter we will examine the functions of the receiving department, discuss inventory theory, and look at the management of hospital inventories.

RECEIVING

The receiving department accepts goods on behalf of the hospital. Once accepted, there is an obligation to pay for the goods. Receiving therefore obligates the hospital for millions of dollars each year. In this section, we will examine the functions and controls necessary to minimize errors.

Receiving Function

The first function of the receiving department is to measure the quantities being delivered and to compare this with both the purchase order and the receipt given to the trucker. This may require counting, weighing, sorting, or the use of some other measurement. As items are counted or measured, the receiving agent should initial the receiving report to fix responsibility for the count. The items are then inspected for damage. This is important because, once the goods are accepted, it is difficult to prove when the damage occurred. The receiving department cannot prove the goods were not damaged on the hospital premises. Damaged items should either not be accepted or the damage should be noted and initialed by the trucker or other carrier.

Often the receiving agent cannot identify equipment, supplies, or other items received because they are of a very technical nature. In these cases, the receiving agent should arrange for an inspection by the user department before accepting anything for which specific technical knowledge is required. The person from the user department should then be required to sign the receiving report.

Deviations in quantity, quality, or specifications should be reported to the purchasing department. Material deviations should be reported before goods are accepted. If a vendor has shipped too much, the hospital can sometimes negotiate a discount rate in lieu of shipping the items back to the vendor.

Copies of the receiving report should be sent immediately to the accounts payable and purchasing departments. Because of the large number of partial shipments, copies required for receiving reports, and other information needs, most receiving departments have a small photocopy machine near the receiving area.

After receipt, goods should be delivered to stores or to the user department as soon as possible. The department should sign for the items. This signature can be on a photocopy of the receiving report.

Many receiving departments have a petty cash fund to pay for collect-on-delivery orders and to pay small freight bills. There should be a dollar limit, set by the chief financial officer, for disbursements from this fund. Petty cash disbursements that exceed this limit can be made from the hospital cashier's fund.

In addition to receiving goods, the receiving department is responsible for shipping bulky items sold or traded in by the hospital. A policy and procedure should be defined to control when items are scrapped, sold, or traded in. This policy should ensure that all retirements of fixed assets be shipped through the receiving dock so that the proper paperwork for fixed asset accounting can be completed.

Receiving Controls

All goods should be received in one place. The hospital should have a policy that defines this centralized function and salespeople should be discouraged from delivering equipment or supplies directly to the user department.

Upon receipt of goods, a receiving report is completed. In most cases, an initialed copy of the packing slip, bill of lading, or other document from the shipper is used as a receiving report. When no other document is available, the receiving agent will fill out a standard hospital receiving report. The form of the receiving report is not important as long as it contains the four essential pieces of information. It should show a description of the items, the quantity received, the date received, and an authorized signature. The receiving report should be included in the hospital's written set of established receiving procedures.

INVENTORY PLANNING

Inventory planning is the quantitative technique used to minimize the hospital's investment in inventories. Inventory control refers to the procedures used to control this investment. Inventory valuation refers to the accounting problems encountered in managing inventories. In this section, we will look at inventory planning.

Objective

The objective of inventory planning is to provide the proper level of inventory at the lowest possible cost. The cost of carrying inventory includes taxes, heating costs, utility costs, depreciation, the cost of equipment to store and handle, insurance premiums, storage expense, janitorial expense, salary expenses associated with handling inventory, record-keeping expense, losses due to obsolescence or deterioration, losses due to theft, and the costs associated with having funds tied up in inventory rather than in some other revenue-producing asset.

The objectives of inventory planning are shown graphically in Figure 11–1. Line A is the cost of carrying inventory. This varies directly with the amount of inventory being stored. In other words, it costs about twice as much to store 200 boxes as it does to store 100 boxes. Line B represents the unit cost of placing an order. This includes the cost of processing the purchase order and receiving the goods and other costs. These costs vary inversely with the size of an order. It takes almost as much money to process an order for 10 items as it does to process an order for 100 items. Line C represents the total costs. This includes the cost of storing inventory as well as the cost of placing an order.

The objective of inventory planning is to find that point on the graph where carrying costs and order-processing costs meet. At this point, the total cost reaches its lowest point.

Figure 11–1 Objective of Inventory Planning

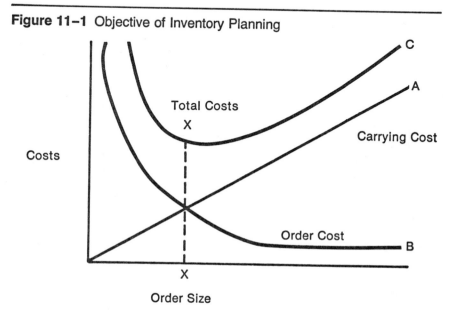

Economic Order Quantity

The economic order quantity (EOQ) is shown in the Figure 11–1 graph as line X. It can be expressed by the following equation:

$$E = \sqrt{\frac{2AP}{S}}$$

where: E = the order size
          A = annual quantity used in units
          P = cost of placing an order
          S = annual cost of carrying one unit in stock
              for one year

The hospital will have to use estimates and approximations in applying the EOQ calculation to items commonly ordered. In performing the calculation, we are measuring the tradeoff between the economics of increased order size and the added cost of carrying additional inventory. Because the hospital must use estimates, an EOQ range should be assumed instead of a point. This range is arrived at intuitively and will be plus or minus a certain number of units.

To illustrate this formula, assume the hospital uses ten thousand units of an item per year. Assume further that the average cost of placing an order is $20 and the cost of carrying one unit in stock for a year would be $1. Our formula is:

$$EOQ = \sqrt{\frac{2AP}{S}}$$

substituting:

$$EOQ = \sqrt{\frac{2\,(10,000)\,(\$20)}{\$1}}$$

$$EOQ = 632.46$$

The hospital should order approximately 650 units each time an order is placed. This is the range in which the sum of the unit cost of storing and the unit cost of placing an order will be lowest.

Quantity discounts also affect unit prices. The above basic formula can be adapted by considering the cost of forgoing the quantity discount and comparing that to the additional storage cost of placing a larger order. Many hospitals use the EOQ equation as a guide and intuitively adjust for quantity discounts as well as other factors that may affect the formula.

Order Timing

The EOQ tells us how many units to order but does not tell us when to place an order. In order to understand when to place an order, we need to make two assumptions. The first assumption is that we can predict with some certainty the time between placing an order and receiving delivery. The second assumption is that usage of the item is constant. That is, there are no high or low points in the demand for the item.

If all of this information were known, the hospital would place an order so that the item would be delivered at the same time the last item is taken from inventory. By timing the delivery to arrive precisely when the item is out of stock, the hospital would minimize its inventory and its storage costs. The number of items in stock is shown graphically in Figure 11–2.

Since orders are delivered when there are no items left in stock, the hospital has the EOQ in stock each time a delivery is made. The reorder point is that level of inventory that will be used up before a shipment arrives from an order if it were placed today. The lead time is the amount of days between placing an order and receiving delivery. If the lead time becomes longer, the reorder point will increase. If the lead time becomes shorter, the amount of items in inventory when an order is placed decreases.

Safety Stock

In determining the reorder point in the preceding example, two assumptions were made. First, we assumed that the time interval between placing an order and receiving delivery could be predicted with accuracy. In reality we cannot predict this time. If the supplier is out of stock, the mail is delayed a day, or the shipment is delayed a day or more because of problems at the point of origin or with the shipping company, delivery will be delayed. The shipment could also arrive ahead of schedule.

Figure 11–2 Level of Inventory over Time

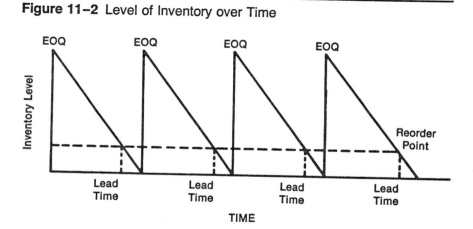

Second, we made the assumption that the usage of this item was constant and predictable. In practice, the demand or usage of an item is not known with certainty. There are times when demand and usage are great and times when the item is seldom used.

Because our two assumptions are not entirely dependable, the hospital can expect to experience times when it is out of stock of an item unless the reorder point is moved back to provide a margin of safety. This margin of safety is commonly known as safety stock.

Before we can determine the level of safety stock for an item, we need to determine the cost of a stockout. The following questions will help to make that determination:

- Can the item be obtained rapidly at a premium cost? Is it available at retail stores?

- How critical is a stockout? Can this affect patient care?

- Can the item be obtained from a nearby hospital with replacement later?

- What substitutes can be used?

These and other questions pertinent to each particular item must be answered in judging the degree of risk.

Once the cost of a stockout is known, the hospital can determine a safety stock level. Instead of ordering so that expected delivery occurs when the inventory is down to zero, the hospital places an order so that expected delivery occurs when the inventory is down to the top of the safety stock level. This is shown graphically in Figure 11–3. Uncertainties of demand and of delivery caused the hospital to go into its safety stock before delivery at points 2 and 4. At point 3 delivery arrived before the hospital reached its safety stock level, and at point 1 delivery was just at the safety stock point.

After the economic order point has been determined and is operating with some degree of accuracy, the hospital may want to adjust seasonally the estimated demand. This would be very time-consuming if done by hand. However, for those hospitals with electronic data-processing capabilities, this enhancement may be beneficial. To seasonally adjust the demand, the hospital must monitor usage of the item by month rather than compute an average monthly usage based upon an annual figure.

The risk of running out of stock does not change proportionally to the size of the safety stock. In other words, if we are 50 percent safe with one thousand items in safety stock, we are not 100 percent safe with two thousand items. It is virtually impossible to protect the hospital from ever being out of stock because demand cannot be precisely predicted. It would take an infinite number of items to ensure that the hospital would never run out. Even the most conservative administrator would not advocate an infinite number of items. The

Figure 11–3 Level of Inventory over Time—Effect of Uncertain Demand

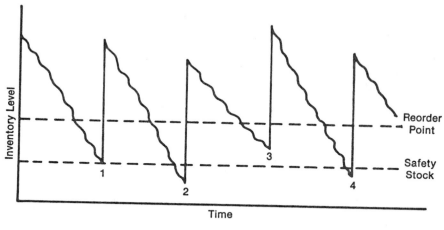

question to determine in computing safety stock levels is not whether or not the hospital should take a risk. The question is, how much of a risk is the hospital willing to assume?

ABC Method of Control

Hospitals perform an extraordinary amount of diverse tests and procedures. The amount of different individual supply items runs into the thousands. Although the principles of EOQ and safety stock should always be kept in mind, the cost of applying these sophisticated control techniques to all items would be prohibitive. Some hospitals divide stock items into subclassifications for purposes of purchasing control. This is done by calculating or estimating total annual purchases for each item and ranking these in descending order. The inventory item on which the hospital spends the most total dollars per year would be at the top of the list. The item on which the hospital spends the least total dollars per year would be at the bottom of the list. This is illustrated in Table 11–1. An actual schedule of inventory items might contain hundreds or even thousands of items.

Now that we have a total annual purchase amount for each inventory item, the items are ranked by categories A, B, and C in descending order by amount of total annual purchases. This is illustrated in Table 11–2.

The final classification of A, B, or C is arbitrary and can be changed from time to time. Those classified A receive the most sophisticated attention. In our example, although A accounts for 81 percent of the purchases, it includes only 10 percent of the items. In this case, the special attention would allow for

Table 11–1 Schedule of Inventory Items

Annual Purchases	Cost Per Unit	Number of Units	Stock Number
$ 500	$ .50	1,000	A–1
20,000	10.00	2,000	B–2
5,000	1.00	5,000	C–3
50,000	5.00	10,000	A–4
10,000	.10	100,000	B–5

frequent ordering but relatively low dollar inventory levels. It would also allow for low safety stock and a plan to expedite purchase orders as well as delivery schedules.

Items classified B receive a moderate amount of attention. One of the methods delineated in the next section might be appropriate in this case. The manner of control will depend upon the hospital, the characteristics of the particular item, and the amount of difficulty in purchasing the item. In our example, B items represent 18 percent of the annual purchases and 18 percent of the items.

Items in the C classification would receive a minimum amount of attention. In this case, inventories might be kept relatively high.

Other Inventory Control Methods

In this section we describe several other inventory controls. These are not intended to be all-inclusive; a list containing all inventory control methods would be endless. The purpose of this section is to show some of the most common techniques and to serve as a foundation on which the creative managers can develop those methods that would work best in their individual hospitals.

The constant order cycle system is a method by which the level of inventory is checked on a regular basis and an order is placed to bring the inventory up

Table 11–2 Ranking of Inventory by Annual Amount

Class	Annual Purchases	%	Number of Items	%	Stock Number
A	$50,000	58	10,000	8	A–4
A	20,000	23	2,000	2	B–2
B	10,000	12	100,000	85	B–5
B	5,000	6	5,000	4	C–3
C	500	1	1,000	1	A–1
	85,500	100	118,000	100	

to a predetermined level. If that level is 5000 units and it is checked on the 10th working day of each month, then on the 10th working day that item would be examined. If the inventory on hand at the time is 1000 units, an order would be placed for 4000 units. With the constant order cycle method, a list can be made of items to check on the 5th working day of each month. Other lists of items can be scheduled for the 10th working day of the month, the 15th working day, and the 20th working day. In this way, the work is spread throughout the month, and a large number of items can be routinely monitored on a monthly basis.

The two-bin system of inventory control utilizes two bins, shelves, or containers. When one bin or shelf is sufficiently empty, inventory is ordered to replace that bin or shelf and the second inventory bin or shelf is used until it is empty. A variation of this technique is called red-line control. A red line is printed on the shelf or bin at a predetermined level. When the red line shows, an order is placed to replenish the inventory.

The order card system is used extensively in retail stores and has been effectively adopted in many hospital storerooms. An order card is placed on the last box or in an envelope behind the last box. When that box is used, the order card is processed to replace the inventory. Another way to use this is to have a permanently placed note on the shelf or wall beneath or behind the last item. This note is a reminder to place an order. The note contains the stock number, vendor name, catalog number, and any other information that would expedite order processing.

INVENTORY CONTROL

Inventories represent a significant portion of a hospital's assets. Because they require a substantial investment, inventories must be efficiently managed. In this section, financial management techniques relating to inventories will be reviewed.

Role of Finance

Although the chief financial officer is not directly responsible for inventory management and control, the amount of money in inventories represents a significant investment for the hospital. The chief financial officer must be familiar with good business practices and ways to control inventories. This will free up funds that can be used more effectively elsewhere in the hospital. Tools for controlling and managing inventories are known and have been tested in non-hospital environments. Many of these tools require computers. Fortunately, most American hospitals either have an in-house computer or purchase computer service on a shared-time basis. The great improvements that have been made in inventory control are available to any financial manager who is willing to take the time to learn about them.

One of the roles of finance is to ensure that the hospital has well-defined inventory management goals. These goals should define acceptance of stockouts, inventory costs, obsolescence, theft, and spoilage. The accounting system should be designed to measure actual performance against the goals. For example, if a hospital is out of stock, what are some reasons for the out-of-stock condition? If a premium price is paid, what caused this?

A final role of the financial manager is the evaluation of goals and objectives. Often a physician or department head will complain to the administrator about an out-of-stock situation. As a result, the administrator will make sure the hospital never runs out of that particular item again, even though this means excessively high inventory levels. Before becoming critical of delayed orders, low stock, or other inventory problems, a study should be made to determine whether the plans were inadequate or were not followed. The study should examine estimates of demand, safety-stock levels, and vendor lead time, and should include a reevaluation of the consequences of being out of stock. This is the essence of effective control and efficient allocation of capital.

Inventory control means managing the investment of funds tied up in inventory in order to reduce losses and keep inventories low. This is a very important aspect of financial management over which the chief financial officer has only indirect control. However, the fact that the control is indirect does not mean it is not critical to the efficient allocation of hospital capital.

Exchange Carts

Exchange carts are widely used in hospitals. They are carts with a predetermined inventory level. Each nursing station or department will have two assigned exchange carts. As one cart is being used the second cart is filled. At the end of a day or other set period of time, the full cart replaces the one being used. The inventory on the partially full cart is then replenished. As this is done, patient charge slips are examined. There should be a patient charge slip for every chargeable item replaced. If there is not, information on the relevant department and day is available for use in correcting the missing charge problem.

Par Levels

Establishing par levels is another acceptable method to control inventory and charge slips. A predetermined inventory is established for each department. At regular intervals, this inventory is inspected and brought back to the par level. Charge slips are collected and compared to the chargeable items missing from inventory. Lost charges are identified quickly and corrective action taken.

Department par levels operate the same as exchange carts. The major difference is that par levels are restocked in the department and kept in a department inventory area. Exchange carts are restocked away from the department, and the inventory is kept on a moveable cart.

Exchange carts are widely used for central supply items because of the volume of use and the large number of items needed. Department par levels are widely used for pharmacy floor stock because of the specialty nature of drugs and the controls required by law over this inventory.

Nonchargeables

A hospital storeroom and pharmacy will issue to departments many items that are not chargeable to patients. Some of these items are office supplies, aspirin, small drug or medical supply items, batteries, chemicals, forms, uniforms, and so on. These should be expensed to the user department.

In order to control these items, nothing should be issued from inventory without a stores requisition signed by a department person on the approved stores list. The requisition is used as a means of calculating the dollar value of items requisitioned each month. The approved list of persons authorized to withdraw items from the storeroom serves as a partial control over the end use of supplies.

Relations with Other Hospitals

Another inventory control technique is concerned with stockouts and the procurement of needed supplies. All critical hospital departments should have a working relationship with one or more other hospitals, even if the nearest hospital is some distance away. This relationship should allow the hospital to borrow drugs, medical supplies, equipment, and other items with replacement at a later date. This relationship should be reciprocal, with one hospital lending items to another hospital when needed. This relationship allows both hospitals to control out-of-stock situations while maintaining a relatively low level of inventory.

INVENTORY VALUATION

A hospital needs a system to enable it to maintain an optimum inventory level. This is not the same as a minimum inventory level. Optimum refers to a system in which reductions are made in inventory only if there are manageable or no stockouts and no significant increase in ordering costs. To accomplish this, the accounting system must produce accurate inventory information. In this section we will examine some inventory accounting concepts.

Periodic versus Perpetual

Inventory valuation methods fall into two broad classifications: periodic inventory recordkeeping and perpetual inventory recordkeeping.

Periodic inventory refers to a method by which inventory is counted and priced periodically. Every time a physical inventory is made, an adjustment is made to match the general ledger amount to the count. The general ledger amount stays at this amount until the next physical inventory. This is normally done once a year. To illustrate, assume dietary inventory is $10,000 on the date of a count. The general ledger is adjusted to show $10,000 for dietary inventory. All food is expensed when purchased, and the inventory account remains unchanged. At the end of a year, another count is made that totals $11,000. Dietary inventory is then adjusted to equal $11,000.

Periodic recordkeeping is used for relatively small inventories that either turn over rapidly or for which the cost of keeping perpetual records is prohibitive. Some hospitals use periodic inventories for dietary supplies, housekeeping supplies, floor stock, and maintenance supplies.

Perpetual inventory refers to a method by which purchases are charged to an inventory account rather than expensed. Withdrawals from inventory are subtracted each month from the inventory account. Thus, a perpetual record is kept of the amount of dollars invested in inventory at all times. Perpetual inventories are kept in those departments or areas that have large dollar amounts in inventories. These inventories may fluctuate significantly from month to month. Areas that normally keep perpetual inventories include pharmacy, central supply, surgery, stores, and sometimes office supplies.

Taking a Physical Inventory

A physical inventory is a count of the items in inventory to determine exactly what is on hand. This total is then compared to the accounting records. If large adjustments are required on a perpetual inventory, this reflects a deficiency in the accounting system, an error in the taking of the physical inventory, theft, obsolescence, or other shrinkage factors. It is not possible to prevent all differences between the general ledger and the actual inventory amounts. Inventory adjustments will always be needed. The hospital's controls should concentrate only on keeping these adjustments manageable and reasonable.

There are nine distinct and important steps in taking a physical count of any hospital inventory:

1. Define the physical existence. In other words, define what to count.
2. Establish control over the movement of inventory.
3. Establish and instruct count teams.

4. Prepare count sheets, tags, or prepunched cards.
5. Count all locations.
6. Clear count areas by a test count or other onsite audit procedure.
7. Clear receiving and establish the inventory in transit count procedures.
8. Apply the lower-of-cost-or-market rule.
9. Extend and foot inventory sheets.

Defining the physical existence means deciding what areas will be included in the physical count. In a for-profit hospital, used linen, floor stock items, and even business office supplies may be counted because this increases the return on equity amount received from Medicare. In a nonprofit hospital, it may be advantageous to include as few items as acceptable in order to expense the items and thereby receive cost reimbursement as quickly as possible.

A good inventory cannot be taken when goods are being added to stock or removed from stock. Before taking a physical inventory, therefore, the storeroom must be closed except for emergency requisitions. Department heads must be informed well in advance to avoid misunderstandings. Local vendors can be asked to withhold deliveries on the day of the count. Receiving should be prepared to keep items received on the dock or other secure area. After the movement of goods through stores has been stopped, the count should be made as quickly as possible.

A count team normally consists of two people. On person calls items and the other writes the number down. It is best if at least one member of the count team is familiar with the items being counted. All plans, instructions, and procedures should be reduced to writing. If they are oral, the auditors will discuss the count with the individuals involved. This is time-consuming and leads to misunderstandings. If the hospital has independent outside auditors, they should be invited to observe the count. If the hospital does not have independent outside auditors, the hospital can invite Medicare auditors to observe the count.

If inventory is taken on sheets, these should be numbered so that all sheets can be accounted for. If tags or computer cards are used, these should be placed in the appropriate stock area. Because the storeroom will be closed during the count, it is important to prepare as much as possible prior to the physical count. In that way stores will remain closed for as short a period of time as possible.

All areas identified at the time the physical existence was defined are counted. Before clearing the area, a sample count or other audit procedure should be performed by either an auditor or another count team. After all inventory has been counted, the hospital should count the items in receiving that were delivered while stores was closed. In addition to items received that day, the hospital may own certain items that are in transit. If title is passed at the point of shipping, the hospital should include these items in its inventory.

The final steps are to apply the lower-of-cost-or-market rule and extend the inventory. The lower of cost or market is explained later in this chapter. Extending the inventory is the process of multiplying the unit cost by the number of units for each item in inventory. The results are then totaled to obtain a total value for the inventory.

Documented audit procedures should be performed throughout the count of an inventory. If the hospital uses independent outside auditors, they should review the audit procedures. If the hospital does not use outside auditors, the chief financial officer should obtain an inventory audit program from a textbook, discussion with other hospitals, or from discussions with auditors. The audit program should be formalized enough to lend credibility as well as to catch discrepancies.

In counting an inventory, controls should not completely verify the inventory figure. The purpose of controls is to establish the reasonableness of the physical inventory count.

Timing Problems

An inventory does not have to be taken on the financial statement cutoff date but should be scheduled close to the fiscal year end. Many hospitals schedule the taking of all inventories a month or two weeks before the year end. Some take inventory piecemeal over several weeks, beginning two months before the fiscal year end. Counting inventories in advance relieves the year-end closing schedule of these tasks.

Because a hospital's normal accounting tracks additions to and withdrawals from inventory, it is not difficult to take an inventory count ahead of time and still arrive at a year-end inventory figure. It is, however, very difficult to take an inventory count after the fiscal year end and arrive at a year-end figure. In this case, special procedures must be used to backdate to the fiscal year end. Because of the difficulty of accounting for inventory after the fact, the physical count should always be scheduled before or on the fiscal year-end date.

Gross Profits Method

The hospital cannot count its inventory every month, yet the monthly financial statements must show a reasonably close value for inventories. For large-volume, fast-moving inventories, most hospitals approximate withdrawals using the gross profits method. Additions to inventory are obtained from accounts payable.

To use the gross profits method the hospital must compute an average markup. This average markup is then used to calculate items coming out of inventory using gross patient revenue. To illustrate, assume a statistical study has shown that the average markup on pharmacy drugs is 225 percent of cost and on central supply items is 250 percent of cost. If gross patient revenue for pharmacy is $100,000 and for central supply is $200,000, drug expense and central supply expense would be calculated as follows:

$$\text{Expense from Inventory} = \frac{\text{Gross Patient Revenue}}{\text{Average Markup}}$$

$$\text{Drug Expense} = \frac{\$100,000}{2.25} = \$44,444$$

$$\text{Central Supply Expense} = \frac{\$200,000}{2.50} = \$80,000$$

Using the above calculation, the hospital would make a journal entry to relieve pharmacy and central supply inventories. In our example this entry would be as follows:

Debit: Drug Expense	$44,444
Debit: Central Supply Expense	80,000
Credit: Pharmacy Inventory	44,444
Credit: Central Supply Inventory	80,000

Pricing Inventory

If prices of goods did not fluctuate, all inventory pricing methods would produce identical values. In periods of fluctuating prices, the hospital must choose an inventory evaluation method that maximizes third party reimbursement and also fairly presents operating results. We will not discuss the theoretical issues of inventory measurement at this point. Rather we will acquaint the reader with some accounting problems through an examination of several different inventory measurement methods. The reader should keep in mind that the only difference between the various methods is in the timing of cost differences.

Specific identification is a method by which all withdrawals from inventory are identified with a specific invoice and charged against inventory at actual cost. Only those items that are very valuable, unique, or easily identified can be specifically identified. Examples of hospital items that may be matched to an invoice when withdrawn from inventory are pacemakers, artificial hips, and other orthopedic implants.

Weighted average is a method of valuing inventory according to a weighted average price paid on several invoices. Weighted average pricing enables the hospital to use a single representative price to apply to inventory items purchased over a period of time. This method is used only with periodic inventories such as those for dietary, floor stock, or housekeeping supplies.

Moving weighted average assigns a single price but with greater weight given to recent purchases. This method is used only with perpetual inventories and is calculated only through electronic data processing. The results obtained are similar to values obtained using first-in, first-out (FIFO) inventory valuation.

FIFO assumes that the oldest units in inventory are used first and that the inventory being maintained represents the most recent purchases. Using FIFO, the ending balance sheet figure approximates replacement cost. However, the objective of matching current expense with current income is not met because items are being expensed out of inventory at a prior-period cost. Income will be highest when prices are rising. This is not a serious problem in hospitals because most major inventory items are turned over in a relatively short period of time.

Last in, first-out (LIFO) assumes the last item in inventory is the first item used. This provides a good matching of current income and current expense because items are expensed out of inventory at the most current price. However, the balance sheet valuation reflects old prices.

To recapitulate, FIFO results in the most accurate balance sheet valuation but overstates net income in periods of rising prices. LIFO results in the most accurate income figure but significantly understates the balance sheet inventory valuation during periods of rising prices.

Last invoice price is widely used in hospitals. This method prices all inventory at the amount on the last invoice. This approximates current replacement values for inventory. From an accounting point of view, there is little theoretical justification for using the last invoice price to value inventory. Moreover, this method reports a low expense because costs are retained in the balance sheet rather than being relieved into the income statement. This delays third-party cost reimbursement. In spite of its theoretical inaccuracy and cost-reimbursement shortcomings, however, last invoice price is widely used by hospitals. The advantages of this method are ease in inventory extensions, lack of extensive recordkeeping requirements, simplicity, and flexibility.

Lower of Cost or Market

Regardless of the method used to price inventory, the hospital should make sure that individual items of inventory are valued at the lower of cost or market. All obsolete items should be removed from the inventory. Items whose value has decreased because of partial obsolescence, aggressive marketing competition, increased production, or some other reason should be written down to their current market value. Market value is a measure of the economic utility of the item on the inventory date. By valuing items at the lower of cost or market, the hospital is measuring and reporting the residual usefulness of the inventory. This results in a more accurate measure of income and expense as well as a more accurate balance sheet valuation of inventory.

SUMMARY

In accepting goods on behalf of the hospital, the receiving department obligates the hospital for millions of dollars each year. It is important that this department carefully count, inspect for damage, and identify all equipment, supplies, and other items before accepting them on behalf of the hospital. Damaged items and other exceptions should be carefully noted. A receiving report is sent to accounts payable and to the purchasing department immediately. After receipt, goods should be delivered to stores or to the user department as soon as possible.

In addition to receiving goods, the receiving department is responsible for shipping bulky items that are sold or traded in by the hospital. An approved policy should define the procedures to be followed when items are scrapped, sold, or traded in.

As the hospital places larger and larger orders, the ordering cost per unit decreases but the cost of holding large inventories increases. By placing small orders, the cost of holding inventories decreases but the ordering cost per unit increases. The point where the savings from holding smaller inventories is exactly offset by the increased costs of placing orders is called the economic order quantity (EOC). At this point, the total cost reaches its lowest point. The hospital will have to use estimates and approximations in applying the EOC point to items commonly ordered.

The EOC tells how many units to order but does not tell when to place an order. The timing depends upon lead time, average usage, and safety-stock assumptions made by the hospital. Lead time is the number of days between placing an order and receiving delivery from the vendor. Average usage is the expected number of items drawn from inventory daily. Neither of these two assumptions can be predicted with certainty, so the hospital maintains a safety stock. Safety stock provides a margin of safety against being out of stock. The risk of running out of stock does not change proportionally to the size of the safety stock. If we are 50 percent safe with one thousand items in safety stock, we cannot assume we are 100 percent safe with two thousand items.

The cost of applying the principles of EOC and other sophisticated control techniques to every item in inventory would be prohibitive. The ABC method ranks items into subclassifications for purchasing control. Low dollar-value items are controlled with relatively less sophisticated techniques. These techniques include constant order cycle, the two-bin system, red-line control, and order card system.

Inventory control means managing the investment of funds tied up in inventory in order to reduce losses and keep inventories low. This is a very important aspect of financial management because it aids in the efficient allocation of capital.

Periodic inventory refers to a method by which inventory is counted and priced periodically with adjustments to the general ledger made only at the time of a physical count. Perpetual inventory refers to a method by which purchases are charged to an inventory account rather than expensed. With this method, withdrawals from inventory are subtracted each month from inventory. Under both methods, a physical inventory count should be made each year. There are nine distinct steps to take in a physical inventory count. Each is important if the results are to be accurate. In taking an inventory, documented audit procedures should be performed. The audit program should be formalized enough to lend credibility as well as to catch discrepancies.

If prices of goods did not fluctuate, all inventory methods would produce identical values. In periods of fluctuating prices, the hospital must choose between several acceptable inventory evaluation methods. The most widely used are specific identification; weighted average; moving weighted average; first-in, first-out (FIFO); last-in, first out (LIFO); and last invoice price. With all of these methods, the individual items of inventory should be valued at the lower of cost or market. Market value measures the residual usefulness of the inventory and results in a more accurate measure of expense as well as a more accurate balance sheet valuation.

DISCUSSION QUESTIONS

1. Name the different steps performed when receiving goods and explain why this function is important.
2. What information should be included on the receiving report?
3. What is the objective of inventory planning?
4. Explain the concept of economic order quantity (EOQ).
5. Define safety stock and reorder point. How are these interrelated?
6. What are some of the costs associated with a stockout that a hospital should consider?
7. Define the ABC method of inventory control.
8. What is the role of finance in inventory control?
9. What is the difference between periodic and perpetual inventory methods?
10. Name the nine distinct steps in a physical inventory count.
11. Briefly define gross profit method, FIFO, LIFO, and last invoice price as these terms are used in inventory pricing.

Chapter 12

Electronic Data Processing

The basic principles of computers are simple. This will become clear as we progress through this chapter. What is difficult to understand is the tremendous speed at which computers operate. Third generation computers calculate in billionths of a second. It would take a person an entire lifetime to do what a large computer can do in a few seconds. It would take an average person four to five minutes to calculate a long division problem. It takes a modern computer less than a thousandth of a second.

The language of electronic data processing (EDP) is unique. Knowing the meaning of many computer terms is often the key to understanding the concepts. The appendix at the end of the chapter is a glossary of commonly used EDP terms. The reader should become familiar with these terms before reading this chapter and refer to the glossary often while reading the text.

WHAT A COMPUTER DOES

The newest and most exciting computer applications in recent years have been to assist the physician in the diagnosis and treatment of disease. The most commonly known application is computer axial tomography (CAT), which takes an x-ray–like picture of a part of the body from several hundred different angles. These pictures are interpreted in the computer memory and used to produce pictures of the body with three-dimensional accuracy. The physician can pinpoint the exact location, size, and shape of a tumor or other disease by looking at pictures of the organ from several different angles.

Another computer application that has been widely used for many years is in reading and interpreting electrocardiograms, which are patterns of heart beats. Analysis of electrocardiograms is difficult and time-consuming, especially for a 12- or 24-hour monitoring. The computer recognizes and points out abnormalities by comparing the patient's heart pattern against normal activity stored in its memory.

Computers are widely used in the diagnosis and treatment of information obtained from a patient's history and symptoms. Information on blood, body chemistry, pain, pulse, heartbeat, and other aspects is fed into a computer that compares it against thousands of case histories stored in its memory. Within seconds, the computer prints out one or more tentative diagnoses with a list of possible treatments and drugs for the physician to consider.

Computers are widely used to monitor patients, perform lab tests, assist in surgery, interpret brain waves and other body functions, monitor prescriptions for drug interactions, and run heart lung machines. Some hospitals are using their computer expertise to perform billing, collection, and other office functions for physicians on a fee basis. This trend will continue as billing becomes more complex.

Use of the hospital computer to assist the medical staff is an important revenue source as well as an effective marketing tool.

Use in Hospitals

Computers have assisted hospitals in the battle against paperwork. Hospitals are probably the most regulated industry in the history of America. New rules and regulations are imposed upon them daily. Without electronic data processing, only the very small hospital would be able to comply with all the regulations. It is becoming increasingly difficult for the small hospital to control paperwork without a computer.

The rest of this section will follow a typical patient from admitting through discharge, billing, and collection in a highly computerized hospital. Few hospitals have all of the computer applications in the narrative. On the other hand, the narrative does not include a complete list of computer applications. Its primary purpose is to inform the reader generally of computer capabilities.

When the doctor informs the hospital of an impending admission, the admitting office initiates a preadmission procedure. The patient is contacted and information is obtained on prior admissions, insurance or other medical coverage, other items that may be needed by billing or collections, allergies, special diets, and so on. The computer automatically searches medical records for prior admissions, accounts receivable for prior payment patterns, and the computer memory for the average length of stay in the hospital for the patient's diagnosis.

Before the patient is admitted, insurance coverage is verified, a bed is assigned for the required length of stay, a medical records file is started, and dietary is informed of any diet restrictions. Pathology, radiology, pharmacy, and other ancillary departments have the physician's preadmitting orders on their work schedule to be completed as instructed by the doctor. This information is all stored in the computer until the patient is actually admitted.

Upon admission, dietary, the business office, medical records, nursing service, and appropriate ancillary departments are all informed automatically. In addition, the patient is listed on the religion census under the appropriate religious preference; on the daily physician census, which is checked by the medical staff; and on the bed census, which prints out by nursing station, medical specialty, and diagnosis.

The physician orders several drugs and diagnostic tests. As the nurse or ward clerk puts these orders into the computer terminal located in the nursing station, several departments' records are updated automatically. If a drug is ordered, a search is made for possible interactions with other drugs, incompatibility with tests to be performed on the patient, and value for the tentative diagnosis. Exceptions are printed in three-level categories by physician. Level-one exceptions are intended to be informative. Level-two exceptions are printed as a warning to the physician. Level-three exceptions cancel the physician's orders. The doctor has the ability to override this cancellation. Drugs and tests accepted by the computer are automatically placed into the patient's medical records, added to the patient's bill, scheduled to be completed by the appropriate ancillary on their daily work schedule, and put into a historical data base for purposes of medical research and medical statistics.

Test results are entered into the computer when known to update medical records and the hospital's historical data base. Many of the tests and procedures performed during the hospital stay are either performed, interpreted, assisted, or made possible through computer technology. The patient stay is carefully monitored on daily management reports. The daily information includes a comparison of estimated length of stay to actual length; a comparison of estimated daily revenue to actual revenue; and daily census reports with gross revenue summaries by doctor, by nursing station, by medical specialty, by diagnosis, and by type of payer. Type of payer includes Medicare, Medicaid, Champus, other government programs, Blue Cross, other major insurance carriers, self-pay, and all others.

At discharge, the patient is presented with a summary bill that provides an estimate of the amount that will be paid by third party payers and the amount due from the patient. If the patient has been classified as a potential payment problem by a patient counselor, a warning is printed for the discharge clerk so that credit and collection can be called to handle the discharge.

Several days after discharge, a final detailed bill, a summary bill, and a special billing are automatically generated. The special billing includes all major programs and insurance companies that require a special form. This may include Medicare, Medicaid, Blue Cross, and other major insurance companies with which the hospital has enough volume to justify setting up and maintaining special billing done by computer.

Until the account receivable is collected or charged off, it is monitored by the computer. Reminder notices, as well as strong collection letters, are sent to patients and third party payers according to a predetermined routine. Because the account appears on a daily reminder list as appropriate, other collection efforts—such as telephone calls, personal letters, and other followup measures— are performed according to schedule. If finally charged off, the bad debt is tabulated by physician, by medical specialty, by primary payer classification, and in any other category deemed important by the credit and collections manager.

Information concerning the patient's stay and collection record is stored in a memory bank. Medical researchers can obtain reports on hospital patients by diagnosis, discharge diagnosis, age, sex, race, and any other criteria captured in the record. These reports may list treatment orders, diagnosis statistics, drug interactions, or patient origin. Administration can order patient-origin studies by zip code, by doctor, by age, or by any other classification deemed appropriate. The controller can order special reports by payer, by physician, specialty, or by any other criteria that would be useful in budgeting or other business functions.

Use with Accounting Reports

In addition to the above applications to aid physicians and hospital departments, the computer also produces many reports designed specifically for accounting. Some of these reports are described in other chapters. In this section, we will outline a few of the more common accounting reports that can be produced by computer.

The working trial balance can be prepared daily, weekly, or monthly. Accounts are not normally merged in this report, even though various combinations are made in the financial statements. The trial balance shows a beginning-of-period amount, debits and credits for the period, and end-of-period balance. Detail for each debit and credit includes a reference to enable the accountant to trace the amount to its source. With the working trial balance, the computer prints an error report. This gives the account number, posting reference, amount, type of error, and computer disposition.

A balance sheet, income statement, source and application-of-funds statement, and fixed asset report compare budget to actual on a monthly basis. This is shown in dollar amounts, in per-patient-day amounts, and in per-procedure amounts. In this way, a comparison of budget to actual can be analyzed completely. Most financial reports show both current period and year-to-date results.

The computer can generate automatically Social Security; workmen's compensation; federal, state, and local withholding; unemployment compensation; and other payroll reports. Budget exception reports can be prepared that report all dollar, statistical, or other predetermined variances over a set limit. This allows the hospital to practice management by exception, with significant savings in personnel time. Cost reports can be prepared monthly in order to estimate contractual adjustments accurately.

Throughout the preparation of the annual budget, computers are used to simulate reimbursement according to different assumptions. This assists the accounting department in pricing strategy, placement of expense in the general ledger, budget decisions, capital budgeting, and long-range planning. Once the annual budget has been approved, computers are invaluable in the preparation of monthly budgets. They can be programmed to calculate historical information by account number broken down into months for the prior year, by weighted average or simple average for prior years, by per-patient day or per-procedure for prior years, or in any other way desired.

Trends and Prospects

The computer applications we have described are like the tip of an iceberg. The applications extend from reminding those on duty to perform a task to asking for verification that the task has been performed. These and other uses of the computer have changed and will continue to change health care delivery in American hospitals. Nursing units, administrative functions, support services, ancillary departments, and physicians are constantly adding to the store of computerized information and receiving responses instantly.

Because of the increasing importance of computers in nonfinancial applications, many hospitals and medical centers are changing their organizational charts so that data processing no longer reports to the chief financial officer. This trend will continue. Finance will always be a major user of the hospital's data processing, but in an integrated system it will no longer dominate.

In addition to performing tasks that cannot be completed by hand, the computer often provides higher quality information than that generated by humans. This is because it is man's basic nature to think and to make decisions in completing tasks. If a function becomes routine and repetitive, there is a high risk of human error. This risk increases with prolonged effort on the same task because of boredom, carelessness, environmental conditions, monotony, and other factors that contribute to mental fatigue. However, the computer never gets tired and remains as accurate at the end of a day as it was in the morning.

HOW A COMPUTER WORKS

Everything a computer does can be broken down into five main steps. These are input, storage, control, processing, and output. In this section we will discuss each of these steps.

Input

Input refers to a medium by which we communicate or talk to the computer. The computer functions in electrical pulses, so a device is needed that converts our thoughts into a form that can produce electrical impulses. Voice transmissions and handwriting have been used experimentally. These have had only limited success, however, because of variations in voice pitch, dialect differences, unique handwriting styles, and other factors that are extremely difficult to program.

For many years, the most widely used input devices were punched cards and punched paper tape. Although these are not as widely used with today's third generation computers, they will be explained because the principles used in more modern input mechanisms are derived from punched cards and punched paper tape.

Information is recorded on cards by punching rectangular holes that represent letters, numbers, and symbols. The cards have 80 vertical lines that are used to record information. The cards have 12 horizontal lines divided into zone punches and digit punches. A number is represented by a single punch in any of the digits. A letter of the alphabet or a symbol is represented by two holes punched in the column. The two holes are a combination of one digit punch and one zone punch.

The 80 vertical lines are divided into fields defined by the programmer. Each field contains a specific unit of information. The size of each field is determined by the maximum length of data that will be entered into it. For example, a card that contains a patient's billing information might be designed as follows:

Columns 1—6	Patient number
Columns 7—26	Patient name
Columns 27—31	Street number
Columns 32—45	Street name
Columns 46—59	City
Columns 60—61	State
Columns 62—66	Zip code
Columns 67—73	Previous month balance
Columns 73—80	Current month balance

This may be keypunched as follows:

623041SMITH__JOSEPH P__
3440__SUMMERSET__DR__NEW__BRUNSWICK__NJ
0122210123740950600

This would be interpreted as follows:

Patient number: 623041
Joseph P. Smith

3440 Summerset Dr.
New Brunswick, New Jersey 01222
Previous Balance: $10,123.74
Current Balance: $9,506.00

The size of the patient name field in this example is larger than needed for the name Joseph P. Smith. In designing the card, the size of the name field was made large enough to contain all of the characters in the largest name in the file.

Often more than 80 columns are needed to complete the record. When this happens, information is abbreviated or codes are assigned to the data. For example, the hospital can assign a three-digit code to represent each doctor on the staff. In this way, even the attending physician with a long name can be added to the patient record with no more than three columns.

Often the information being created in the file cannot be condensed to 80 columns even with abbreviations and codes. This would be the case when a patient is admitted. In this case, two or more cards may be needed. The first one or two fields of each card can designate the card in the series, and fields can be designed for each card.

The computer reads the holes in the punched cards with metal brushes or with photoelectric cells. A hole completes a circuit, and an absence of a hole means a circuit is broken. Each item of information is called a bit. The bits together form computer words that are a series of electric pulses.

Punched paper tape operates the same way as cards. Since it uses fewer columns, it must string many lines of information together. As the punched paper tape is read by the computer, fields of information are created by electrical impulses. Paper tape punches can be economically produced as a result of some other operation. A paper punch can be added to accounting machines, calculating machines, typewriters, cash registers, and other office equipment. As hospital employees perform their normal routine functions, a machine readable tape can be produced as byproduct at little additional cost. This eliminates the need to keypunch the information later. A great disadvantage of punched paper tape is its slow transmission speed. Even if one uses seven- or eight-channel tape, transmission speeds of only 150 characters per second is considered good.

Other equipment used by hospitals for recording data in machine sensible language includes magnetic ink inscribers and perforators. Magnetic ink in characters that are optically read by electronic data-processing equipment has been used successfully for patient charge slips. The patient number is imprinted from a charge plate, and the ancillary department imprints the procedure number. The procedure number tells the computer the name of the department and the name of the test. If charges are automatically priced by the computer, the patient number and procedure number are all that is required.

Perforated coupons are prepared by machines that perforate and print at the same time. This application is used primarily in installment books, but it could also be set up to record a series of outpatient visits, to record statistical data such as meals served by nursing station, or for time cards.

All of the input devices discussed up to this point must be converted into an electromagnetic medium before being processed by the computer. Conversion can be off-line, which means peripheral equipment separate from the computer, or on-line, which means equipment that is an extension of the computer. The advantage of off-line equipment is that it does not tie up expensive computer time. Whether on-line or off-line, conversion to an electromagnetic medium is relatively slow.

The trend in hospitals today is toward entry into an electromagnetic medium. Fields are defined on magnetized tapes, disks, or drums for entry at high speed into the central processing unit of the computer. The principles applicable to punch cards and punched paper tape also apply to tapes, disks, and drums. A spot on the tape corresponds to a column on a punched card. The spot is either on or off. It is either magnetized or not magnetized. The magnetized and unmagnetized spots are read and interpreted by the computer.

Many computers have a time-sharing or time-allocation program. This allows information to be transmitted, edited, and accepted directly into the computer. Third generation computers operate in billionths of a second. A data-entry operator would be taking up expensive computer time if everything on the computer were stopped in order to accept information. With a time-allocation program, data are entered into a buffer or holding zone. The computer time-allocation program waits until there is sufficient data and then takes the data out of the holding zone for processing at high speed. The advantages of direct access into the computer are high speed and the availability of editing routines.

Editing routines decide whether the information being entered is appropriate for the data being processed. They then check on the validity and accuracy of the data. Good data are accepted and data that does not pass all of the validity and other editing tests are rejected with an error message. Editing can be performed by a minicomputer with the information transmitted later to the main processing unit. This transmission is called core-to-core because it is a direct communication between the core storage of one computer to the core storage of another computer.

Data entry into an electromagnetic medium can be accomplished by use of a keyboard similar to a typewriter, by use of a cathode ray tube and keyboard, by pushing buttons or labels in a predetermined sequence, by placing cards in slots, or by using other devices. The telephone is used to request and receive computer information as well as to enter data. The buttons on the modern telephone make an excellent small key punch station.

Modern technology has made it possible for input devices to be as close as a few feet to as far away as thousands of miles from the computer without loss of quality and with little loss of time. Data are generated over dedicated telephone lines, via satellite, onto tapes for shipping to the computer site, and by direct wire hookup to the computer. Shared service companies often are thousands of miles from the hospital they service yet provide service that is as efficient and as timely as if it were from an inhouse computer. The principles and techniques used to input data are the same for all kinds of computer processing.

Storage

Data that are stored in the memory unit of the computer are in primary storage. Data that are stored on tapes, disks, and other devices and connected to the computer as needed are in secondary storage. The use of secondary storage increases the capacity of the computer to process because with a system of storage and retrieval the computer's memory becomes infinite. The computer can be programmed to store and retrieve information as needed.

There are two basic kinds of information that need to be stored. They are instructions and data. Instructions tell the computer how to perform, and data are the information to be worked on. The problems of and documentation necessary to perform the storage function of electronic data processing are illustrated in the following example.

Assume the computer operator wishes to update the accounts receivable file. Before the computer can start on the update, it must have direct access to the program that tells it what to do and how to do it. Each command to the computer is represented by a separate set of instructions. The required program is loaded into the memory of the computer. Once this program is stored, the task of processing data can begin.

The data to be processed are obtained and loaded on the computer. These data include yesterday's accounts receivable information, room-and-board charges generated today, ancillary charges generated today, other charges and payments made today, recognized contractual allowances, and today's bad debt writeoffs. Current charges are added to yesterday's balances. Then payments, contractual allowances, and bad debts are subtracted from the balances, and a new accounts receivable detail and balance is created. The new information is printed on a report, and today's information is stored until update time tomorrow.

Controls over the storage and use of the data in storage cannot be too strong. Almost without exception, the most expensive, time-consuming data-processing errors are on data tapes. Some examples of these errors will clarify how critical the problem can be. In some cases, the wrong day's balances are updated with today's information in a process that does not save today's input, or the error is not discovered until today's input is erased. The hospital is left with a worthless update and no immediate way to solve the problem. In another example an operator might mistakenly erase today's balances instead of the balances from two days ago. The problem here is that today's balances can be updated only with yesterday's transactions, not two days ago.

Sometimes an error in a program change will erase or erroneously alter data. For this reason, many hospitals will never run a new or revised program on current data unless a backup tape or disk exists. If a program is destroyed, it can be rewritten. However, if data are destroyed, they cannot always be completely reproduced, even at great expense.

Control Unit

The control unit is one of the most important parts of an electronic computer. The control unit receives instructions from the computer's stored programs. The programs stored in the computer are said to be in primary storage.

The control unit selects the order to be used in performing the various steps in the program, the path the data will follow, and where the information should be stored in memory. The control unit of a computer tells the input device what to put into the computer and when to do it, and it tells the output device when and what to print or transmit. The control unit properly connects all of the units of data so that the process is completed properly. This unit also watches over the operation as a whole to ascertain that every step is performed in the proper sequence and on time.

The control unit of a computer has been compared to the chef in a large restaurant, to a traffic cop at a busy intersection, to the control tower at an airport, and to the referee at a sporting event.

Central Processing Unit

Although the central processing unit or brain of the computer has the mentality of a newborn infant, it can perform computations that a thousand Ph.D.s working together as a team could not perform. This is possible because the computer can follow even the most complicated and tedious instructions without error. Whatever we tell a computer to do, it will do. Consider the problem of solving the following by hand: $(6981462456 \div 3787321593498)^4$. How to solve this could be explained rather quickly, but it would take well over a half an hour to perform mentally the long division and to calculate the quotient to the fourth power. And there would be a good chance of making a mistake. A computer, however, could solve this problem in a fraction of a second and be 100 percent accurate. This does not mean the computer is smarter than humans, who can drive cars, generate original thought, interpret emotions and body language, plan for the future, learn from the past, and so on. A computer can only do what it is programmed to do. It is not capable of original thought, of making original choices, or of performing any other original feat of intelligence.

The computer works on an on-off, yes-no principle. A resister is either conducting or not conducting; voltage is either present or not present in a circuit; a spot on a tape, drum, or disk is either polarized or not polarized; a postion on a card either has or does not have a hole. Following this yes-no principle, most computers use a binary number system. This means that instead of the ten digits on which our system of mathematics is based, a computer has only two digits. In our calculations, we start at zero, and when we reach nine we start all over again with zero, but now we put a one in front of the first column, then a two, and so on. When a computer gets to the second digit, it starts all over again with another column. A comparison of binary and decimal numbers is shown in Table 12–1.

The symbols for 0 and 1 are the same in both systems. The binary system does not have a 2, so one is created by moving to a new column position. A 2 in this system therefore becomes 10. In the decimal system, each time a power

---

Table 12–1 Decimal versus Binary Numbers

Decimal	Binary
0	0
1	1
2	10
3	11
4	100
5	101
6	110
7	111
8	1000
9	1001
10	1010
11	1011
12	1100
13	1101
14	1110
15	1111
16	10000
17	10001
18	10010
19	10011
20	10100
21	10101
22	10110
23	10111
24	11000
25	11001

of 10 is reached (10, 100, 1000), a new column is started. In the binary system, each time a power of 2 is reached (2, 4, 8, 16), a new column to the left is started. The size of the numbers does not slow the computer down because it operates in billionths of a second.

Because the computer cannot generate even the simplest thought by itself, a computer programmer must prepare a set of detailed instructions. These instructions are a series of codes that open or close an electrical circuit. These circuit codes are called a computer program. The program details each small step needed to solve a problem. There is no such thing as an insignificant detail; the computer is not capable of making even seemingly insignificant assumptions.

The machine language of a modern computer consists of thousands of circuits, and the instructions must be written in binary numbers. To program in machine language, the programmer would have to remember every circuit, every memory position, and every routine in the computer. This would entail so much detail that even the most talented programmer could write only simple routines. The machine manufacturers, therefore, publish an assembly language with each computer model.

The assembly language is composed of what is called mnemonic codes. These codes consist of letters, numbers, and symbols that stand for routines in the computer. The computer uses a program in its primary storage to translate the assembly language instructions into binary codes. Assembly language, although many times simpler than machine language, is still difficult to learn.

An entire series of higher level languages have been developed that resemble English or mathematics as we know them. When programming (which can also be called coding) is done in a higher level language, a compiler is needed to translate this into machine language. A single statement in a high level language can produce the compilation of a series of instructions. In assembly language, one symbol can produce only one routine or instruction. Some of the more common higher level programs are COBOL, FORTRAN, and PL1.

COBAL is an acronym for Common Business Oriented Language. This computer language closely resembles English and enables those who do not understand the more complex computer languages to learn quickly to write instructions to the computer. The compiler takes the instructions written in COBOL and prepares a machine language, a binary set of instructions. COBOL is used in a hospital's business applications.

FORTRAN is an acronym for Formula Translation. FORTRAN is used primarily to solve mathematical and scientific problems. It is used extensively in the hospital's medical and technical applications.

PL1 is an acronym for Programming Language 1. The program was developed to combine the advantages of COBAL and FORTRAN. Because PL1 was developed with scientific as well as business applications in mind, it can be used effectively for both types of programming.

COBOL, FORTRAN, and PL1 are by far the most commonly used programs in hospitals today. However, many other high language programs are used with lesser frequency.

In summary, it can be said that a computer works in a simple technique called on-off. Because the computer can understand only this simple principle, all instructions must be broken down into a seemingly infinite number of components. To make this possible, the programmer solves the problem in a series of pyramid-like steps. First the solution or set of instructions is broken down into parts and coded in a common language. The compiler then takes these instructions, breaks them down into many more parts, and converts them into machine language. The machine then carries out the instructions in a binary system process that may require many circuits for each instruction.

Output

Output devices have been defined as computer devices designed to translate electrical impulses representing data processed by the central processing unit into an intelligible and persentable format. What this means is simply that an output device enables the computer to share its solution to a problem. The output device may be a magnetic tape, a magnetic disk, a drum, a set of punched cards, a printer, the core of another computer, a set of instructions to a machine or instrument, photoelectric film, or some other device.

The output device may be next to the computer, thousands of miles from the computer, with the input device, or entirely separate from the input device. With modern technology, it is no longer necessary to concern ourselves with problems pertaining to the placement of the computer in relation to input and output devices.

The most widely used output device is a printer. The printer can print a bill, a report, a letter, or a message. It can produce a graph or simulate a picture. Printers may use an inked ribbon or may burn letters on special paper with electrical impulses. However, the printer is relatively slow compared to other output mechanisms.

Another well-known output device is the cathode ray tube, often called a CRT. This operates like a television set and can be equipped with a device to produce a paper (hard) copy of whatever is on the screen. The limitation of a cathode ray tube is that it can produce only one page of information at a time.

Computers can be made to produce an image on either a microfilm or a microfiche film. This image is exactly like a picture from a camera. Instead of creating the image from light, the film is etched with electric current. The process is extremely fast, and the film is sent for processing as if it had been produced on a microfilm machine.

Output can also be placed on a magnetic tape, magnetic disk, or drum or onto the core of another computer. These devices are used when the information is needed to process a subsequent report or will only be read by humans using a CRT or other visual display machine.

CONTROLS

The trend in hospital data processing has been toward larger, more integrated systems. Data entered in one department are automatically interfaced with data in other departments and with subsystems in other functions. All of this is performed with lightning speed. As this trend spreads, the need for input controls becomes increasingly more important because mistakes become more difficult to correct, especially if not corrected immediately.

Program Documentation

Documentation should begin when programming is in the planning stages and should be carried on throughout the time the program is being used. Lack of adequate documentation is a major problem in hospitals when changes need to be made or when researching the reasons for program errors. Following are some of the items that should be contained in a program documentation file for every program used by the hospital:

- Copies of card layouts and form design drafts.
- Preprogramming flow charts. These include input data and their sources and sample output designs. These flow charts should be supported by a complete narrative; and if the program calls for detailed calculations, these calculations should be shown.
- Programming sheets. These include the program language, copies of all the coding, copies of all the programs as actually listed by the computer, and copies of the program input as keypunched.
- Copies of all testing procedures, test run data, and results.
- A complete copy of the program run manual, which details all of the steps the computer operator must follow to run the program on the computer.
- System changes, evaluation studies, copies of actual output, and any other data pertinent to the program.

If the hospital is using a shared service, some of the actual programming flow charting and coding will not be available. However, documentation on input, operating procedures, system flow charts, output, and maintenance should still be kept in a file created for each program.

The chief executive officer or the chief financial officer should either personally audit data-processing documentation files or delegate this to others with periodic review. When a person in data processing leaves the hospital, it should be an easy matter for someone unfamiliar with the program to answer questions or to make modifications in it.

Operating Schedules

A hospital data-processing department cannot run efficiently without adherence to strict scheduling. The first phase of scheduling should set times when input data are due in the data-processing department. The time for keypunching or other data entry; program-run times, including an estimated number of minutes each program will take on the computer; tentative rerun times if needed; and the time of day output is due in the user department should all be documented.

In the master time schedule for data processing, time should be set aside for new program debugging, running special requests, and system maintenance. Without this scheduling, special requests and program debugging either never get done or are performed at times that disrupt normal operations.

Input-Output Controls

All computer input should be logged and compared to output. The amount of detail logged and compared must be designed to fit the needs and output of the individual hospital. If the hospital logs too much detail, much of the savings generated through use of the computer will be used to keep logs and to control data. If the controls are not adequate, erroneous or incomplete data may be accepted by the computer with no way of identifying the source of the error.

Control totals are manually added by batch of input and placed on a control sheet. These totals are compared to the batch totals printed by the computer. Sometimes a field of input is totaled and audited for purposes of verification even though these totals are not needed in the application of the program. These are called hash totals. Hash totals are normally used only for important columns of information, such as employee numbers in payroll.

If any of the totals on the input control sheet do not agree with the total accepted by the computer, the difference should be entered in a corrections register. Amounts in the corrections register should be carefully monitored until they are reentered and completely accepted by the computer. Sometimes a line of data will be reentered several times before it is accepted.

KINDS OF COMPUTER APPLICATIONS

The choice of a computer or computer service is one of the most important decisions a hospital can make. All of the different computer systems cannot be covered in this section. Instead, some of the major differences will be outlined to enable the reader to understand the complexity of the problem.

Digital versus Analog Computers

There are two kinds of computers: analog and digital. Analog computers measure while digital computers count.

The name *analog* is derived from the word *analogous,* which means similar. Analog computers register changes in voltage, resistance, linear distance, or shaft rotation to measure the proportional changes in two numbers. Problems are solved by creating an analogy in the computer and then measuring the results. Analog computers are used for specialized business problems and for scientific applications. In a hospital, they would be used in nonbusiness areas.

Digital computers use combinations of data to solve problems according to a set of programmed instructions. Digital computers are used in all regular financial applications. The operating principles of digital computers were discussed earlier in the chapter.

In-House versus Shared Service

An in-house computer is one that is owned or leased and under the control of the hospital. The hospital is responsible for the equipment, insurance, and normal maintenance as well as programming and implementation of changes. The advantages of an in-house system are flexibility and sometimes lower cost. Flexibility is especially important to large hospitals because computers seem to evolve characters that are unique to the operations of a particular institution. Shared services tend to be inflexible in programming and often cannot respond adequately to the special needs of a larger hospital.

A shared service is an arrangement in which the hospital has input and output devices at the hospital to send and receive data from a computer that is owned and operated by a company that sells processing services. The computer is often located hundreds of miles from the hospital. There are several advantages to using a shared service. Programming changes, such as those in payroll withholding tables at the beginning of the year, are done automatically. All of the problems of scheduling the computer, of breakdowns, and of maintenance are removed. Except for the lack of flexibility, shared services usually offer excellent programs, and the format of the output often meets management needs.

Other Computer Services

In addition to in-house or shared systems, there are several other computer services the hospital can use. These services can be used for special projects, specific applications, or, in a smaller hospital, as the entire electronic data-processing option.

Block time may be purchased from another company in the area. Often firms will be willing to rent a portion of their excess computer time. Usually the block of time offered is after normal working hours. The rates are very favorable because the firm is selling time that they already have but are not using. In this case, the hospital is required to write all of its own programs, to provide trained computer operators, and to function as if it had an in-house computer. A firm selling block time does not provide any assistance. If the hospital wants to purchase excess computer time, the chief financial officer should ask bankers, board members, and other associates who may have excess time available. In large cities, the classified section of the newspaper may have ads offering computer time for rent.

Service bureaus and banks are another important source of computer service. Service bureaus normally contract to perform a computer service. Banks normally contract to perform a specific specialized function. The service is usually acceptable and the cost reasonable. There are two major disadvantages to a service bureau. The first is that they usually perform one or two functions but cannot handle all of the hospital's data-processing needs.

Some hospitals use a service bureau for their accounts payable or general ledger functions. Many banks offer payroll services at a reasonable rate. This allows them to take advantage of a payroll check float as well as to utilize excess computer time. There are several nationally known appraisal companies that will process all of the hospital's fixed assets. This includes additions, retirements, depreciation schedules for Medicare and Medicaid, and computation of Medicare gain or loss on disposal of assets. The reports produced by these companies are widely accepted by Medicare intermediaries.

Minicomputers are another option that hospitals have used. Technology advances have made minicomputers small, reliable, less expensive, and flexible. Minicomputers can be purchased and programmed to perform applications in inventory control, accounts payable, fixed assets, and numerous other hospital functions.

PLANNING FOR NEW APPLICATIONS

If the hospital substitutes faster and more advanced computer systems without proper planning, the results will probably not be satisfactory. Personnel costs will multiply, and scheduling problems will destroy the effectiveness of the computer. This occurs because merely substituting equipment is a job-orientation approach, whereas, to be effective, the planning for such changes must involve a systems approach.

Need for Feasibility Studies

Although the powers of a computer are considerable, there are costs to consider in setting up and maintaining a computer application. A feasibility study is a means of surveying and evaluating the advantages as well as the costs and other disadvantages of using a computer.

A feasibility study should begin with an analysis of the proposed benefits. These benefits generally fall into three categories: (1) reduction in clerical costs, (2) development of information that may be too time-consuming or too costly to obtain manually, and (3) introduction of modern management techniques to enable administration to run the hospital more effectively. Many hospitals carefully study the first of these but neglect the second and third. It is not unusual to find a careful economic study that indicates that a computer system will cost as much or more than the present manual system. However, if it develops better management information or introduces better business techniques, it may be beneficial to approve the higher expenditure.

Data-processing applications normally cut across organizational and functional lines. To achieve a successful application, personnel in several areas of the hospital must have adequate input and must understand the overall benefits to the hospital. If the hospital is considering a major application, an outside consultant should be called in to coordinate the feasibility study and summarize the results.

In contracting with a consulting firm to perform a feasibility study, the hospital should make sure the persons who will conduct the study have actual operating experience. Many consultants have excellent credentials and extensive auditing, consulting, or teaching experience, but only limited operating experience. Because of the extent to which organizational and functional lines will be crossed, operating experience is necessary.

The Feasibility Study

The first step in a feasibility study is the selection of a study team. The members of the study team should be employees who have the time and the interest to serve. The study team should also possess the required skills to understand all of management's policies, plans, and procedures. The first duty of the team is to define a charter that sets forth the purpose, timetable, and objectives of the study. If the members of the team are not from diverse areas of the hospital, the report may not take all affected functions into consideration.

Once the study team has defined its charter, an analysis of the present system is undertaken. This is usually done by interviewing employees successively in line with the information flow that will be converted to the new system. The interview schedule usually begins with the supervisor. This interview provides an understanding of the broad picture and is used to solicit cooperation and support. Detailed information is then obtained from the personnel doing the work. Copies of reports, forms, and other information are obtained. All functions are listed with estimates of volume, the machines required, their costs, and personnel time requirements. The accuracy of this information is verified with the supervisor, and differences in understanding between the supervisor and the employees are resolved. An estimate of the present cost of each operation is prepared. This estimate covers personnel, equipment, maintenance, and supplies.

As the present cost is determined, an analysis is made of present costs that can be eliminated. This analysis should include not only present costs but also a projection of anticipated future costs with documented future volume estimates.

The documentation of the present system serves as a basis for determining the proposed system's specifications. The documentation should assess (1) output, (2) files to be maintained, (3) flow of information, and (4) scheduling.

Output includes all of the information that will be required and the frequency of the reports. The actual format of the reports is not defined at this time, but all of the information needs are documented. The files to be maintained should include enough data to satisfy special requests and potential future information needs. The input forms will need to be changed to satisfy the information-on-file needs of the new computer application. The flow of information will include many new policies and procedures that must be approved by top management. Approval of these new policies and procedures should be obtained early in the feasibility study. If agreement cannot be obtained, the flow of information should be altered until the required policies and procedures are acceptable. The last specification of the proposed system to be defined is scheduling. The new computer application should be capable of meeting or improving the timing of information released with the present system. The proposed schedule should consider existing reports and proposed new reports.

After the specifications of the proposed system are defined, consideration of alternative hardware and software can begin. This begins with an evaluation of proposals from manufacturers, service bureaus, in-house data-processing personnel, and shared-service representatives. If proposals from several firms are received, it is best to schedule these presentations on the same day. In that way, the members of the study team are committed to only one day, and, because the proposals are all fresh in the minds of the study team, comparability between them is enhanced.

For major systems changes, one or more members of the study team should make site visits to other hospitals to evaluate equipment, schedules, costs, implementation problems, and other factors. If consultants have been hired to coordinate the feasibility study, they should accompany hospital representatives on these site visits. A copy of the report on each site visit should be given to each member of the study team.

The final step in a feasibility study is the determination of costs. Personnel costs should cover supervision, programmers, operators, and clerical employees. In developing an estimate of clerical salaries, care must be taken to include all new functions. Some of these new functions might include control clerks, scheduling clerks, magnetic tape librarians, and distribution of reports. Nonpersonnel costs include costs of supplies, utilities, paper, ribbons, magnetic tapes and disks, small equipment, insurance, and so on.

The last element of expense is computer costs. Whether the hospital is considering an in-house system or a shared service, computer costs will be very difficult to determine. There are two reasons for this. The first is that processing times on the computer can only be guessed at. Estimates from salespeople are usually inaccurate, but the hospital has little other information available. The second reason is the difficulty of developing costs for nonproductive time and special applications. Nonproductive time includes time for reruns, setup, program editing, input and output difficulties, and peripheral equipment breakdowns. To compensate for these unknowns, it is best to be very liberal in estimating computer time. This will make the projected savings of the proposed new system seem conservative but will probably prove to be more accurate.

Evaluation Score Sheet

Because of the many diverse criteria that must be evaluated, many feasibility study teams use an evaluation score sheet as a tool in the decision process. The use of an evaluation score sheet lends objectivity to the selection process and provides a definitive explanation to management for the final recommendations. To use this technique, the study team should first define comparative criteria. These may have to do with implementation costs and schedules, the quality of support from manufacturer or service company, cost evaluations, available backup equipment, delivery schedules, compatibility with present EDP equipment, processing time, flexibility to meet future requirements, the availability of present programs, and adaptability of programs. After the criteria have been defined, the study team should assign weights to each criterion to measure the relative importance of the various factors. The assigning of weights is a subjective process, but with active team input it can be very reliable.

An example of a computer evaluation score sheet is shown in Table 12–2. On this score sheet, five proposals are compared. Three of the proposals are for an in-house computer system and two are for a shared service. Based upon the comparative criteria and the assigned weights, proposal D for one of the shared services is the best alternative, and proposal E for the other shared service is the second best alternative. In an actual evaluation of a new computer system, there would of course be much more than eight judgment criteria. However, the principles illustrated would be identical.

IMPLEMENTING THE SYSTEM

Once a decision on a new computer system, a new application on an old system, or a change in a computer application has been made, a plan must be formulated for implementation. This plan should include nine tasks:

1. training and education of personnel
2. designing the system and programming
3. developing charts and schedules for implementation of the system
4. preparation of the computer site and wiring for peripheral equipment
5. program and system testing
6. parallel testing
7. conversion of major files
8. reorganization
9. post implementation evaluation.

The personnel to be trained includes operators, programmers, systems analysts, clerical personnel, and personnel in the user departments. The degree of difficulty encountered in this educational process will depend on the individual

---

Table 12–2 Computer Evaluation Score Sheet

Comparative Criteria	Assigned Weight	In-house			Shared	
		A	B	C	D	E
1. Report of on-site visit to other hospitals	10	10	8	8	7	9
2. Installation costs	5	1	4	3	4	4
3. Flexibility to needs	20	17	15	18	20	14
4. Monthly operating costs	15	13	12	13	11	11
5. Fit with proposed system specifications	15	14	14	14	12	11
6. Support personnel availability	10	8	7	8	9	9
7. Backup equipment availability	15	6	8	7	15	15
8. Ongoing operating costs	10	8	9	8	7	7
Total points	100	77	77	79	85	80

personnel and their adaptability to change. In order for the new system to be successful, this part of the implementation schedule must involve as many people as possible early in the conversion.

The designing of the system and programming start with the source documents and end with the education of user personnel in how to use the output of the system. Site preparation will be concerned with space requirements, flooring, wiring, air conditioning, power installations, and the move to the new site. Any peripheral equipment, such as CRT devices in user departments, should be considered. The designing of charts and schedules for implementation may include a pert chart or other time sequence chart.

The individual programs or other components of the system are tested and debugged, first individually and then in the aggregate. The entire system undergoes a final complete testing in the parallel testing stage. In parallel tests, both the old and the new system are processed and their output compared. This ensures the accuracy of the new system. Although the initial basic plan is refined and changed throughout the different steps in the implementation, it is during the testing phases that most changes are made. These phases include program testing, system testing, and parallel testing.

Conversion of major files should be accomplished as soon in the planning as possible. Whenever possible, data files should be converted prior to actual installation of the computer, using specific equipment for that purpose. During the conversion, records and totals should be checked for discrepancies so that a completely accurate new file can be set up.

With data processing cutting across organizational and functional lines, work flow and assignments will change. Some departments will experience a significant drop in man-hour requirements, while others may experience a significant increase. This may necessitate a new organizational structure or a reassignment of personnel. Reorganization requirements normally become apparent in the postimplementation evaluation of the system. This evaluation determines the success of the conversion. During this phase, forecasted implementation schedules are compared to actual schedules, costs savings are verified, budgeted startup costs are compared to actual costs, and an operational audit of the system's effectiveness is performed.

SUMMARY

The basic principles of electronic data processing are simple. What is awesome and hard to understand is the tremendous speed with which computers operate. Modern computers calculate in billionths of a second. Most hospitals use computers every day to assist physicians and to win the battle against paperwork and also in accounting and financial applications.

In a highly computerized hospital, the computer system is highly integrated and automatically ties many departments together. A highly integrated system begins with preadmission. The system assists in admission, schedules routine as well as special doctor orders, tracks ancillary activity as well as housekeeping, dietary, and nursing services. In addition, medical records and billing are automatically updated. At discharge, a summary bill is generated, and the patient's bill is automatically followed until it is paid in full or written off.

Computers generate better accounting reports than those generated by hand because the computer does not suffer from fatigue. Everything that a computer does can be broken down into five main steps. These are input, storage, control, processing, and output. Input refers to the medium in which electrical pulses are sent into the computer. For many years punched cards were the predominate input mechanisms in hospitals. The trend today is toward direct entry into an electromagnetic medium. With timesharing and editing programs, direct on-line entry into the computer has become common.

There are two basic kinds of information stored in a computer: instructions and data. This information can be put in either primary or secondary storage. Primary storage is in the core of the computer. Secondary storage is apart from the computer. The control unit of a computer selects the order to be used in performing the steps of a program, the path the data will follow, and the data to be stored in memory. The control unit acts as a guide to the central processing unit. Most central processing units operate on an on-off principle. A spot, resister, circuit, or other device is either magnetized or not magnetized. Because of the simple on-off principle, computer language must use a binary number system.

An output device receives output or processed information from the computer. In addition to operating with a printer, computers can operate CRTs, record on magnetic tapes or other magnetic devices, produce film images, and control machinery.

As hospitals use larger, more integrated data-processing systems, controls are becoming increasingly more important. These controls include program documentation, operating schedules, and input and output controls. They are necessary in shared-service applications as well as in in-house computer systems. In addition to in-house and shared-service companies, a hospital can obtain computer services in other ways, for example, by purchasing block time or mini computers or from service bureaus.

New systems or changes to an existing computer system require a feasibility study. For substantial changes, an independent outside consulting firm is often hired to coordinate the feasibility study and to summarize the results. Steps in a feasibility study include selection of a study team, definition of the study-team charter, analysis of the present system, determination of the specifications for the proposed new system, consideration of hardware and software, and completion of a cost study.

Because of the many diverse criteria that must be evaluated, many feasibility study teams use an evaluation score sheet. The use of an evaluation score sheet lends objectivity to the selection process.

Implementing a new computer system requires extensive planning in order to be effective. There are nine specific tasks involved in a good conversion program.

DISCUSSION QUESTIONS

1. Outline some ways in which electronic data processing can assist the hospital's preadmission program.
2. How can the computer be used to reduce lost charges from ancillary departments?
3. Comment on whether the data processing department should report to the chief financial officer on the organizational chart.
4. What does an EDP input device do?
5. What are the advantages of magnetic tapes and disks as input devices over the traditional punched card or punched paper tape?
6. Explain how a timesharing or time-allocation program works on a third generation computer.
7. What is the difference between primary storage and secondary storage in a computer?
8. What role does the control unit of an electronic computer play?
9. Explain the difference between the binary number system and the decimal number system.
10. What is contained in a good program documentation file for any hospital program?
11. What is the purpose of input and output controls on information processed by data processing?
12. Compare and contrast in-house versus shared-service computer systems.
13. Describe briefly a feasibility study for a new computer application.

Glossary

This glossary of commonly used electronic data-processing terms is not intended to be all-inclusive or even representative of the most often used terms. The intent is rather to present the basic concepts of electronic data processing in American hospitals in nontechnical language and an informative style.

Alphameric. A term used to describe data that contain both alphabetic and numeric characters.

Analog computer. A computer that simulates measurements by electronic means, for example, by varying voltages.

Audit trail. A means of tracing data back to original source data.

Batch processing. A system of processing a number of similar items in groups.

Batch totals. The sum of a column of input used later to verify data.

Binary system. A numbering system that has only two digits, 0 and 1. The binary system is used by digital computers.

Buffer. That part of a computer system that temporarily stores information until the computer system processes it.

Bug. An error in the program or in the system.

Central processing unit. That part of the computer that carries out the instructions and solves the programs given to the computer.

Character. One of the digits, letters, or other symbols that are recognized by a computer.

COBOL. Acronym for Common Business Oriented Language. A computer language widely used in business operations.

Coding. Using symbols and abbreviations to give instructions to the computer. Synonymous with writing the program.

Collating. Combining of data from two or more files into sequence in one file.

Compiler. The program that converts the instructions written by the programmer into instructions that can be interpreted by the computer.

Computer operator. The person in a computer system who manually controls the operations of the computer.

Control total. The sum taken on a particular field in a group of records to be used for checking program, machine, or input reliability.

Control unit. A major part of the computer that directs the step-by-step instructions given to a computer and that oversees the scheduling of the operations called for by the program.

CRT. Acronym for cathode ray tube, which is a television-like device used to display or store data.

Data file. A major unit of information that is stored. Examples of data files include accounts receivable, payroll master file, and general ledger.

Debugging. Identifying and correcting errors in a computer system or program.

Destructive readin. A process of putting new data into a file in which data previously stored is destroyed in the update.

Digital computer. A computer that processes data by combinations of digits.

Disk pack. A device that contains a set of magnetized disks.

Editing. The process of deciding what data to accept, examining them for accuracy, and rejecting those that do not meet predetermined parameters.

Electronic data processing. The processing of data and calculating of results by an electronic machine, such as a computer.

Field. A group of consecutive columns of data used for a specific purpose.

File maintenance. The periodic modification of a file to include changes that have occurred.

First generation computer. A class of computers that used vacuum tubes.

Flowchart. A graphic portrayal of a sequence of operations, an accumulation of data, or the steps used to solve a problem.

FORTRAN. Acronym for Formula Translation. A computer language widely used in scientific and engineering applications.

GIGO. Acronym for garbage in, garbage out. A commonly used term meaning that the quality of the computer output cannot be better than the quality of the input.

Hardware. The equipment and other machine devices in a computer system.

Hash totals. The sum of numbers of a specific field. Used for verifying purposes.

Input. Data entered into a computer system for processing.

Installation. A particular computer system and its overall process.

Machine language. A system of instructions written in a binary code of electronic impulses that are used to direct the computer.

Magnetic tape. A tape that has been coded with a magnetizable material. Used to record information in the form of polarized spots.

Memory. A device on which data can be stored for retrieval at a later time.

Mnemonic. A contraction or abbreviation used to represent the full expression.

Nondestructive readout. A process in which data are read out of storage repeatedly without being destroyed.

Operation manual. A manual that gives detailed instructions to a computer operator on how to complete a job.

Peripheral equipment. Equipment that is not under the direct control of the computer, such as a printer, card reader, or cathode ray tube.

Primary storage. Storage in the main storage area of the computer itself.

Procedure. A predetermined way to accomplish a given task.

Programming. The advance preparation of instructions for use by the computer.

Random access. A storage device by which access time in retrieval is made to be independent of the location of data or sequence of input.

Real time. Processing of data instantaneously as they are received, enabling the user to have immediate control.

Second generation computer. A computer that uses transistors and operates in millionths of a second.

Secondary storage. Storage on magnetic tapes, disks, drums, or other devices that are not directly connected to the computer.

Simulation. A representation in a computer program of a real model in order to mirror the effects of changes in the model. Used to determine the probable effects of changes in assumptions.

Software. The programs and documentation of a computer system.

Source document. Original paper from which information regarding a transaction is recorded.

Subsystem. An identifiable portion of a main system.

Terminals. Devices for input and output that are some distance from the computer. They are often connected to the computer by telephone lines.

Third generation computer. A computer characterized by miniaturization and great speed. Operates in billionths of a second.

Chapter 13

Fixed Assets

The purpose of this chapter is to consolidate all of the financial considerations relating to the acquisition of capital assets by a hospital. These begin with a venture analysis, which is the financial justification and approval, and continue through the acquisition period until the fixed assets are recorded in the accounting records and depreciation begins.

CAPITAL BUDGETING

There are an almost infinite number of capital expenditures that a hospital can make each year. There seems to be no end to the race for new medical technology. Capital budgeting is the process of allocating limited capital funds for the most appropriate expenditures.

Institutional Goals and Objectives

A good capital budget process is one that does the most to help the hospital achieve its goals and objectives. A hospital that has not defined its long-range goals and objectives cannot have a good budget process.

In most industries, capital budget decisions are relatively easy to make. Any corporate finance book will explain how to use such techniques as net present value, rate of return on investment, other discounted cash flow methods, and profit impact considerations. In hospitals, especially nonprofit hospitals, capital decisions are more difficult. They cannot be ranked according to rate of return and subjected to sensitivity analysis. Hospital capital budget decisions are ranked according to their support of the hospital's goals. This will become increasingly more important in the future as hospital funds become less abundant.

A long-range plan has two main parts that are relevant to capital budgeting. The first is the choice of major objectives. Is the hospital striving to become a major referral hospital with several centers of excellence, such as heart surgery, renal transplants, or neonatal intensive care? Is the hospital a good community hospital that refers the more acute patient to another hospital? Will the hospital stay at its present size, or will there be a major expansion? Once the board has decided upon the hospital image or major qualitative objectives, major budget decisions can be made to support this. An excellent community hospital would not consider expensive, highly specialized equipment; and a major referral center would consider only highly specialized equipment that supported one of its defined centers of excellence.

Once the major objectives have been decided upon, they must be detailed into subobjectives. The subobjectives define programs and time periods for the achievement of the programs. It is important that the long-range plan be formalized. Both the objectives and the subobjectives should be put into writing, and a financial plan to achieve these objectives should be developed. Tradeoffs between objectives may be necessary. Therefore, the plan must be updated annually.

Department Requests

Once institutional goals and objectives have been defined and communicated to department heads, the capital budget process can begin. Two kinds of capital budgets are developed. The first is a long-range budget; the second is a current year budget.

The long-range capital budget will include only large expenditures. Most hospitals try to budget all expenditures forecasted to cost $100,000 or more. Because of the effects of inflation, some hospitals attempt to budget all expenditures that are expected to exceed $75,000. In this way, the hospital can make a substantial error in predicting price inflation and still be able to go ahead with all expenditures that exceed $100,000. The format for a long-range capital budget request for Community Hospital is shown in Exhibit 13–1.

The amounts are requested in columns for each year of the five-year request. This facilitates organizing and summarizing the data by year. It also facilitates making tradeoffs between years.

As the departments are preparing five-year requests for items expected to exceed a certain dollar limit, the chief financial officer should prepare an estimate of the annual expenditures for items less than the limit. This estimate is prepared in total for the entire hospital. It can be forecasted by extending the trend developed from historical data from the past few years, by computing a ratio of normal capital expenditures to equipment depreciation and extending this ratio to estimates of future depreciation expense, by a study of fixed assets records to determine how many assets are expected to expire according to the assigned accounting life, or by some other method.

Exhibit 13–1 Community Hospital Five-Year Capital Budget Request

Description of Project	RIA*	19X0	19X1	19X2	19X3	19X4

Expenditures over $75,000

In Thousands

Submitted by _____

Department _____

*R=Replace, I=Improve, A=Add

As the long-range capital budget is approved, department heads should clearly understand that this approval is tentative. Changes in the projected availability of funds, failure to get an approval for the certificate-of-need application, changes in the hospital's goals, and new advances in medical technology could all negate a tentatively approved capital expenditure.

The current year budget request should include all department capital needs regardless of their dollar amount. These should be ranked by department heads in descending order of importance and labeled as urgent, essential, or desirable. Strict definitions of urgent, essential, and desirable should be developed by the hospital to ensure uniform use of these terms. Because of a tendency to overrank budget request items, the accounting department will have to work with department heads every year to gain acceptance of the terms in the budget process. Desirable items will be labeled essential and essential items will be labeled urgent by zealous departments hoping to improve the chances of approval for their requests.

In addition to ranking their requests, departments should identify each line item of their current year request as being an addition, as a replacement of existing equipment or facilities, or as an improvement to existing fixed assets. A short narrative describing the request and showing how the items support the hospital's goals for the year should also be supplied. This information will be used by administration and the budget committee to approve or reject budget requests. One person should be assigned to review the narratives of all departments for clarity and completeness. This person will act as a resource person to assist any department with its request. This is to prevent the approval of capital budget requests from only the more articulate department heads.

The last piece of information needed on a current year budget request is the expected month of payment. This information should not be used in the approval process. However, the month of payment is needed to complete the cash budget. In the chapter on cash budgeting there is a schedule for balance sheet items. The purchase of fixed assets is a balance sheet item in the cash budget.

The date of the proposed capital expenditure should not enter into the approval decision-making process. Once the total expected cash available for capital expenditures is known, the hospital decides which capital requests can be approved. The timing of the availability of cash is not important to this decision. Temporary borrowing, short-term financing, and other methods are used to solve availability of cash problems.

Approval Process

There are always more capital requests than the hospital can afford. This is a predictable occurrence every year. The processes used to evaluate and pass on these requests vary widely from hospital to hospital, depending upon the management style of administration, the perceived or real needs of the medical staff, and the nature of the board of trustees. This section will examine some of the philosophical thought processes that should be considered in capital budgeting and will briefly outline several advanced analytical techniques that can be used.

Since there are always alternative uses for the money to be spent on capital purchases, we can conclude that there is a value or cost that can be assigned to money. This cost is expressed as either a loss of borrowing power or a loss of investment opportunity in other assets.

If the hospital has existing debt, cash used to purchase fixed assets could be used to reduce that debt if the purchase is not made. If additional borrowing is used to purchase fixed assets, it will reduce the borrowing power available for future projects that would bring a benefit to the hospital. Unless the hospital is totally debt free, there is some cost attributable to the loss of borrowing power every time a capital asset is purchased.

If the hospital is fortunate enough to be debt-free, there is still a cost of capital that can be attributed to each fixed asset purchase. This is measured as a reduction of the availability of funds to invest in inventories, prepaid assets, accounts receivable, or securities. Since investment in inventories, prepaid assets, and accounts receivable is difficult to quantify, the cost of capital is usually shown as the loss of investment opportunities in securities. The expected rate of interest available on securities in which the hospital normally invests is known and can be assigned as the cost of capital. The chief use of this is to set a floor below which any investment in fixed assets will be unattractive.

Once the hospital has assumed a cost of capital based upon either loss of borrowing power or loss of investment opportunities, all capital projects can be ranked in order of their value to the hospital as expansion projects, cost-saving projects, or defensive and maintenance projects. This ranking can be done by estimating net present value, by estimating the ability to attract physicians' use of other services, by estimating cost savings, or by some other logical method. A comparison of the different ranking logics that can be employed is beyond the scope of this book. However, in the remainder of this section, we will outline several advanced analytical techniques that can be used in capital budgeting.

Sensitivity analysis is a way of showing how expenditure values may be affected by changes in the assumptions used. The analysis is usually presented in graphic or tabular form to illustrate how much net value of the expenditure will differ from the estimate if physician satisfaction, patient demand, anticipated cost savings, the labor rate, or some other assumption does not come out as expected. Sensitivity analysis does not estimate an assumption's probability of outcome. It shows rather a variety of alternative values so that administration can determine the impact of a range of possibilities.

Linear programming is a mathematical analytical technique that is used when there is a need to select the best combination of capital expenditures and there are definite limits on one or more of the factors involved. When a decision to invest in a given capital expenditure is based upon its net present value, the choice of equipment, or the combination of equipment, the expenditure's profitability might be based on linear programming analysis. Outside consultants, such as certified public accounting firms, are often needed to carry out linear programming studies; but less specialized accountants and analysts can identify opportunities for these studies and assist in carrying them out.

Simulation and modeling have a wide variety of uses in capital budgeting. Simulation is a process of using one or more trial runs of a mathematical model to learn about its possible outcomes. Then a forecast model is developed that simulates an outcome that is representative of expected real outcomes. Simulation is especially useful where the major assumptions may be expected to take on various patterns of variations and it is impossible to settle on single values for estimating purposes.

Risk analysis in capital budgeting extends sensitivity analysis by attaching probability factors to estimates of cost, revenue, and other assumptions. Calculations of the likelihood of possible results can then be made. Many hospitals use simple forms of risk analysis without calling it by that term. A project estimate that shows a high, middle, and low figure is an example of risk analysis. Another example would be an analysis that shows an optimistic result and a pessimistic result. Risk analysis gives administration an opportunity to judge the risk element in a decision.

It is important to note that capital budget rankings or analytical techniques do not replace judgment. They can, however, present meaningful information to administration so that judgments can be made of the risks, the tangible and intangible benefits, and the need for capital items that have been approved.

Evaluation of Leasing

Leasing is a form of purchase that can be used for almost any capital purchase. In this section, we will discuss some of the factors that make a lease attractive to a hospital, compared to a capital purchase.

Often someone has special skills or special purchasing power that can be obtained more economically through leasing than through purchasing. This may be the case when a hospital leases through a local taxing authority that issues bonds to finance purchases. Interest earned on bonds issued by a taxing authority is exempt from most state and federal income taxes and, therefore, will attract a much lower interest rate than bonds issued directly by the hospital. Economies may also result through leasing because the owner or lessor has the ability to purchase and maintain a large number of similar installations more efficiently than individual hospitals. Another advantage of leasing is the ability to transfer the risk of future operating cost increases to the lessor. The hospital can negotiate a fixed lease expense over the life of the lease, while the owner assumes all the risk of maintenance cost increases, material cost increases, and other cost increases. When the owner assumes additional risks, the monthly lease payments increase.

Another reason for leasing is that it gives the hospital an ability to use an asset for less than its useful life and then dispose of the asset without having to sell it. There are several circumstances that would make this desirable. One is that, in a field of rapidly changing technology, leasing can be an important hedge against obsolescence. Another circumstance might involve a diagnostic mechanism that may or may not be accepted by the medical staff. It may be desirable to lease such equipment for a period of time and monitor its use by the physicians. If it is a success, a longer lease or outright ownership can be undertaken.

The best known reason for leasing is as a source of available capital. A hospital can obtain through leasing the use of large sums of money that may be unavailable from other financing mechanisms or available only at high interest rates. Often a lessor and the hospital will agree in advance on the exact terms of the lease and will execute a formal lease. The lessor then will use the lease as collateral in securing a loan to finance the purchase of the lease property. If the lessor can obtain more favorable interest rates than the hospital or if the hospital wishes to save its borrowing power for a future anticipated purchase, this arrangement works to the benefit of both the lessor and the hospital.

Sometimes leasing is the only alternative. The lessor may be a computer or manufacturing company that wishes to protect its technology. In such cases, the owner may simply refuse to sell at a reasonable price, and leasing may be the only practical way to acquire use of the property.

VENTURE ANALYSIS

Hospitals cannot afford to go into new programs and commit extensive resources without in-depth planning. Without such planning, the result would be chaos, bankruptcy, or both. The problem of evaluating new equipment and programs can be broken down to three major categories. These are (1) justification of need, (2) ability to operate, and (3) ability to staff. Whatever form an individual hospital's venture analysis takes, it should be concerned with these three aspects.

Justification of Need

The equipment or program being proposed should be defined in a manner that relates the expenditure to the objectives of the hospital. This definition should explain how the objectives of the proposal are both attainable and justifiable on the basis of five specific criteria. If the objectives of the new piece of equipment are neither attainable nor justifiable in light of these criteria, the project should be aborted. The five criteria are:

1. Can the hospital afford this?
2. Can the necessary training of personnel be accomplished within a reasonable time frame?
3. Does the community need it?
4. Can the hospital market the service?
5. Is the demand strong enough to warrant the purchase?

After the program has passed these objective tests, the hospital can be sure of its need. The next step is to evaluate the politics of obtaining a certificate of need, if the project cost requires such a certificate. The hospital should attempt to determine the health planners' views on the proposed expenditure and its effect on areawide cooperation or competition between and among hospitals. If the expenditure will help to attract staff physicians or favorably influence the costs of the hospital, this should be noted in the certificate of need. If the expenditure will adversely affect the costs of other area facilities, the hospital should prepare a defense against this in the certificate of need. If the service is needed but beyond the ability of the hospital to acquire, the possibility of helping another hospital initiate and carry out the program can be examined. Helping another hospital to acquire a new program with either direct or indirect assistance is an excellent way to attract important favorable support for the hospital's existing programs.

Justification of need includes carefully designing and defining the requirements of the program. Most new equipment becomes obsolete for the hospital before it is worn out. The economic life and the residual value thus should be estimated. What other alternatives exist to achieve the proposed program objectives? These would include options available to patients as well as options available to staff physicians. If the hospital is considering a capital expenditure to replace a piece of equipment, it should define the actual deficiencies of the present service. Often the deficiencies are not as real as they seem, and the available money can be used for other projects.

The last consideration in justifying the need for a new service is to describe its teaching value for staff physicians, hospital employees, teaching programs affiliated with the hospital, and for others. Equipment which has a high teaching value often increases the utilization of other hospital resources.

Ability To Operate

The ability-to-operate category of a venture analysis study concerns primarily the financial implication. In planning the finances, the accounting department should first seek information available from other hospitals regarding costs and revenue for other hospitals. Often the salesperson can assist in locating other facilities that have had experience in operating the program that the hospital is considering. Government, philanthropic support, and grants are available for many projects if the hospital investigates these possibilities. If the hospital simply cannot afford a needed piece of equipment, the pros and cons of joint ownership with a physician or hospital group can be studied. Many hospitals have entered into agreements whereby physicians purchase equipment and receive part of the revenue from its use.

A new service can be financed by loans, through leasing, or by diverting present resources. In planning the finances, it is important to plan projected start-up costs and operating costs in addition to the purchase price. The continuing costs of a service that are most often overlooked include the additional costs of maintenance, housekeeping, nursing, and other support departments. Direct operating costs must include wages and supplies in addition to depreciation or lease expense.

A two-year cash flow analysis for a new service includes many assumptions. Some of these assumptions are estimated occasions of service, proposed charge structure, bad debt assumptions, contractual adjustment assumptions, and collection time lag by type of third party payer. Once a program is implemented, the hospital should have a plan to evaluate actual results against planned results. Were the additional personnel and capital needs precipitated by the program according to plan? How close is the actual revenue to budgeted revenue, and what are some of the reasons for major variances? The best way by which a hospital can improve its forecasting techniques is to monitor carefully actual results against forecasts.

Ability To Staff

The third element of a feasibility analysis is the determination of the hospital's ability to staff the new service. If the present medical staff is not qualified to administer the new technology, a physician recruitment program must be undertaken. The success of recruitment efforts is difficult to predict. If a specialist must be recruited to the staff in a relatively short period of time, the hospital should consider contracting with a recruiting firm.

The nonphysician direct personnel needs must also be identified and the funding for their salaries in the startup phase determined. Many new ventures take well over a year before they become self-supporting. In setting prices, the projected loss of a new service is often supported by raising prices in a stable identifiable present service.

Direct personnel needs can be met through recruitment or by transferring existing personnel. Both of these alternatives will require specialized training as the new service is started. In addition, the increased demands that will be placed upon support departments must be considered. Housekeeping will need to clean the new area, maintenance must heat and cool the space, and nursing and other ancillaries may experience additional demands. If these are not well planned and documented before a new service is initiated, the hospital may be faced with a financial drain that it cannot afford.

FIXED ASSET ACCOUNTING

Accounting for fixed assets in hospitals is becoming increasingly important. This is partly because of the requirements of third-party cost reports such as Medicare and Medicaid. Fixed asset records are also important for insurance purposes. This is especially true with the increasing involvement and responsibility of boards of trustees.

Recordkeeping

There is a minimum amount of basic information that should be found in all good property records. This is true of computer-assisted property records as well as those kept by hand on cards or in ledgers. The first piece of necessary information is a tag number that identifies a particular item. It is best to affix on the asset a plate or other identifying mark with the tag number. The next important piece of information is the location of the asset. This always includes the department. If the hospital has several buildings, it will also include a code for the building where the asset is located.

The date of acquisition must be in the records. This date is important in determining the depreciation status of the property and in calculating loss in disposition of assets. If may be helpful also to have a code that indicates the kind of transaction used to put the asset in the department. For example, there may be separate transaction codes for purchase, exchange, transfer, build, and major repair.

The description of the asset should be complete enough in the records to fully identify the asset. For each piece of machinery that has a serial number, the number should be a part of the description in the property records. Color, dimensions, brand name, and the kind of material (i.e., wood, metal, plastic) used to make the asset are all useful items of information in the description. The original cost, estimated useful life, and accumulated depreciation make up the balance of the basic information required in all good fixed asset records. Many hospitals include more information than we have described. This is especially true for those hospitals with sophisticated computer systems to record and track property records.

Equipment and other items are constantly being transferred to another department, retired, traded in, or otherwise disposed of. Therefore, it is important for the hospital to have a periodic fixed asset inventory. Fixed asset inventories should be taken every two or three years. This is accomplished by providing each department with a list of all assets assigned to that department. This list is then compared to all assets actually located in the department. Assets on the list that are no longer in the department are crossed off, and the department head is required to indicate, if possible, what happened to the asset. Items that are in the department but not on the fixed asset list must be added. The department should indicate how this asset was acquired. Was it purchased, transferred from another department, or constructed? Once the physical inventory has been taken and compared with the accounting records, the differences must be reconciled.

Outside Contractors

If the hospital has an expansion or other major construction program that will be performed by an outside contractor, there will be a contract that describes the construction and legally binds the contractor and the hospital to perform several things. In this section, we will briefly examine several aspects of a contract with an outside contractor that must be considered.

The payment clause determines how the contractor will be paid. This clause will normally provide for partial payments based upon estimates of percentage of completion. The hospital must make sure the contract defines who will determine the percentage of completion. It should be an engineer independent of the contractor. The hospital should also make sure the contract provides for a retained payment. If the construction is 50 percent completed, the contractor should be entitled to receive substantially less than 50 percent. The retainage is for two reasons. The first is that if the contractor pulls out of the job and leaves, it will cost extra money to have another contractor come in to finish the project. The second reason for a retainage clause is to guarantee acceptable performance by the contractor. The last installment of the retainer should not be due until the work has been accepted.

Most contractors will attempt to negotiate one or more escalation clauses into the construction contract. These can cover raw materials, labor, subcontractors, or other items and are designed to protect the contractor against unforeseen cost increases. If the risk of inflation is transferred to the hospital, the dollar amount of the contract should decrease. If the contractors assume this risk, they should have a larger profit built into the contract price to compensate for it. The hospital should make sure the contractor can never recover all of his cost increases through escalation. This would create a situation in which the contractor had no incentive to hold costs down. It is easier to let costs escalate freely than to attempt to control them. Unless the contractor shares some of the cost increases with the hospital, there will be no incentive to do anything to control costs. It is cautioned that whenever a contract calls for reimbursement of a portion of the contractor's costs, the administrative and accounting costs of enforcing the contract increase tremendously.

It is important that the contract require the contractor to provide a list of all major component parts used in construction. This inventory of components should be detailed enough to enable the accounting department easily to identify and record the component parts when the project is completed.

The engineering and maintenance staffs should be involved in the clause that defines the recordkeeping required of the contractor. These records become the source used to order replacement parts, to assist in maintenance requirements, and to assist in repair troubleshooting.

The audit clause gives the hospital or its agent the right to examine the contractor's accounting records. An audit clause should be part of any contract that has an escalation clause or cost-plus clause of any kind. Unless audit procedures are agreed to in the beginning, the contracting firm may be reluctant to allow the hospital to examine its records. The audit clause should also define how applicable overhead will be determined and verified; what kind of documents, such as original cancelled invoices and copies of checks, are acceptable; and what recordkeeping requirements are required to be met by the contractor.

It is not unusual for the contractor to insist that the audit be performed only by an independent certified public accountant acceptable to both parties.

The hospital can require a performance bond or other assurance that the contractor is financially as well as technically capable of performing under the contract. If the contractor became bankrupt, could not obtain working capital financing, or could not afford to pay for damages resulting from off-specification work, the hospital could suffer severe financial losses. Provision for these contingencies should be agreed upon in advance.

The insurance clause defines who is responsible for insurance covering fire, vandalism, personal injury liability on the construction site, damage from storms and other natural occurrences, and workmen's compensation. This clause will also define the minimum dollar amounts of coverage for each of the different kinds of insurance, stipulate acceptable insurance companies, and specify the loss payee. The provision should also require proof of insurance for all coverage that must be obtained by the contractor and define what is meant by acceptable proof of insurance.

The hospital and the contractor may find it advantageous to include some type of termination clause in the contract. This is called force majeure in most contracts. It provides for termination of the contract as a result of occurrences that are beyond the control of both parties. The clause will define occurrences and provide for the manner in which the contractor will be compensated. The hospital may also wish to provide for termination of the contract in the event the contractor goes bankrupt. The liabilities of the hospital when a contract is terminated through contractor bankruptcy should be carefully defined in order to avoid litigation that may delay completion of construction.

The last important clause of any construction contract is the arbitration clause. This clause provides for settlement of disputes in specified areas that may become subject to dispute. With an arbitration clause, the hospital can ensure that disputes involving technical matters are settled by experts rather than by a judge who is untrained in the particular field. Arbitration clauses are also used to avoid lengthy and costly legal battles. Many arbitration clauses provide for each party to appoint an independent arbitrator. The two chosen arbitrators would then select a third arbitrator to complete the panel. The three arbitrators would then decide on an equitable solution. The award made by the panel would be binding on both the hospital and the contractor.

Work Order Files

At the beginning of a large construction project, the accounting department should anticipate and prepare for closing out the work-in-process accounts and for establishing permanent fixed asset records. This is accomplished by establishing a work order file for each portion of the construction that has accounting significance. The work order files then become the source of accounting journal entries as well as the source for establishing detailed asset records.

The work order files will contain all invoices, records of payment, correspondence, and other documentation pertaining to a major segment of the construction. On a large addition to a hospital, a work order file would be established for each of the following segments: architecture, electrical, plumbing, heating and air conditioning, roofing, elevator and escalators, building shell, interior decorating, financing fees, fixtures, and equipment. These work order files may also contain copies of construction-change orders that have been approved by both the hospital and the contractor. Construction-change orders are prepared to provide for additions or deletions from the original contract or for changes in specifications and to authorize substitutions.

Basically, the work order files are a tool used to organize a large construction project into smaller parts. They can be used to divide the accounting work as well as to make the recordkeeping manageable. Work order files can be used for in-house construction projects as well as for construction performed by outside contractors.

In-House Construction

When a construction project or major remodeling is undertaken by the hospital's own work force, all the controls and other problems that are normally covered by a contract must be done internally. The first of the problems is control over expenditures. The work by the carpenters, plumbers, and others already in the department will be charged to normal maintenance department activity unless controls are established to charge it to the construction job. Applicable fringe benefits must also be charged to the job. A common way to accomplish this is to use time sheets. Supplies must also be carefully monitored to make sure that the hospital knows the cost of the construction project. The hospital already maintains a substantial stock of materials, supplies, and other assets that will become part of the in-house construction. Withdrawal slips charging items to the construction project should be completed for all items drawn from stock.

Costs of in-house construction projects are controlled through the work order. The work order authorizing in-house construction should be almost as complete as an outside construction contract. The work order should include detailed estimates of cost by major category. These categories include labor, materials, supplies, subcontracting, and other items. The work order should also include a detailed description of the asset with appropriate specifications. Finally the work order should set target dates for completion of each phase of construction and indicate who is authorized to approve expenditure of monies in connection with the work order.

Change Orders

Construction change orders are common occurrences for both outside-contractor and in-house construction projects. Some hospitals have extensive approval and control procedures over original project approval, yet do not even monitor change orders. This can result in embarrassing cost overruns.

There are two kinds of construction change orders. The first is a change order that alters the specifications or due dates. Most of these will not require any additional money, and they can be approved by the project manager. If the alteration or new due date will require additional funds, an approval process must be established. This approval process must address both the additional money for the immediate change and any accumulative additional money required. For example, on a large construction project, the project manager might be given authority to approve change orders for up to $5,000 to an accumulated total of $100,000. Additional approval would be required for a change order that will cost more than $5,000 in additional funds. Additional approval would also be required for any change, regardless of the dollar amount, after the project director has approved $100,000 in additional costs.

The other type of construction change order is one that adds to the original scope of the project. Add-on change orders should ideally be subjected to the same approval process as the original project. If the add-on is relatively minor, many hospitals require only administrative approval. It is important to control carefully add-on changes in order to control costs and to ensure that the completed construction will not inadvertently alter the scope of the project.

Other Fixed Asset Accounting

Other fixed-asset accounting problems include retirements, transfers, and preventive maintenance programs. Procedures should be established to account properly for each of these.

Retirement of fixed assets can occur through trade-in, sale, or scrapping of the equipment, building, or other asset. An approval process is necessary for retirements. The process should provide at least as much control as the approval process for acquisition of assets. When an asset is traded in, the approval process should ensure that the trade-in allowance has been negotiated and is as high as possible. If the trade-in allowance is significantly less than market value, the hospital should consider selling the asset rather than trading it in. On trade-ins, the approval form is used to calculate gain or loss on retirement of the asset, to add any remaining book value to the price of the new asset for depreciation, and to remove the asset from the hospital's detailed records.

Transfers of fixed assets must be recorded in accounting in order to change depreciation records as well as to account for the physical existence of the equipment. It is not uncommon for items such as desks, file cabinets, calculators, typewriters, and other items that are commonly used by all departments to be transferred several times in one year. Unless a transfer form is completed and sent to accounting, control over these assets will be lost.

Preventive maintenance programs are a requirement of the Joint Commission on Accreditation of Hospitals (JCAH). In addition to the JCAH requirement, preventive maintenance programs can be cost justified. Since the accounting records include all pieces of equipment used, many hospitals are tying their preventive maintenance monitoring into the accounting records. This is especially useful if the fixed asset records are highly automated on a computer. The computer program would then have all preventive maintenance and testing dates in its memory by tag number. On the specified date, a message would be printed telling the department head that it is time to perform preventive maintenance or to perform retesting of a piece of equipment. The computer could also be programmed to verify by input that the applicable maintenance or testing has been done and to keep a complete history by tag number of all maintenance performed on the equipment.

SUMMARY

There are three major questions that must be answered in any venture analysis program. These are justification of need, ability to operate, and ability to staff. Justification of need relates the project to the objectives of the hospital, addresses the issue of certificate of need, and explores the possibility of obtaining the new program in cooperation with other hospitals. Justification of need also completely defines the new project. Ability to operate is concerned primarily with the financial implications. This aspect requires a feasibility study, proforma statements of income and expense, and a cash flow analysis. Ability to staff involves a determination of physician availability and availability of other required hospital personnel.

Hospitals can make an almost infinite number of capital expenditures each year but have limited funds. A good capital budget process is one that does the most to further the hospital's progress toward its stated goals. If the hospital does not have established long-range goals, these should be defined by the board of trustees before the capital budget process is begun.

Each year, the hospital should prepare two capital budgets. The first is a long-range capital budget that includes only large departmental expenditures. The second is a current year budget that is more definitive. Current year budget requests should be classified by department heads as urgent, essential, or desirable. The department heads should also indicate whether the item being requested is a replacement, an improvement, or a new addition. All narrative justifications for requested capital items should be reviewed by one person in order to prevent the possibility of approving only those capital budget requests from the more articulate department heads.

Because the hospital has alternative uses for every dollar spent on capital purchases, it can be shown that there is a present value or cost that can be assigned to money. Ranking capital requests in order of their estimated worth or value to the hospital is the first phase of capital budgeting. This may be followed by sensitivity analysis, linear programming techniques, simulation modeling, and risk analysis.

Leasing may be selected as an alternative to purchase for nonfinancial as well as financial reasons. Some of the nonfinancial reasons include the opportunity to acquire special skills, the ability to abandon the asset before its useful life expires, and the use of the lease as a hedge against obsolescence. In some cases, leasing may be the only practical alternative.

When the hospital negotiates a construction contract, there are important clauses that must be negotiated involving payment, cost escalation, record-keeping requirements, audits, performance bond and insurance requirements, termination of the contract, and arbitration. Whether the construction project is to be performed in-house or by an outside contractor, the accounting department should establish work order files to accumulate all the required information.

DISCUSSION QUESTIONS

1. For a hospital venture analysis program, briefly define justification of need, ability to operate, and ability to staff.
2. How can capital budgeting be used to further the hospital's progress toward its long-range goals?
3. Compare and contrast a hospital long-range budget with a short-range or current-period budget.
4. How can sensitivity analysis, linear programming, and simulation models be used in the capital budgeting process?
5. What are some reasons why leasing is often a better alternative than purchase of an asset?
6. What basic information is found in all good hospital fixed asset detail records?
7. Explain the basic steps in planning, taking, and following up on a hospital physical inventory of fixed assets.
8. What is the purpose of work order files in a construction project?
9. What controls are needed on construction change orders? Why?
10. How can fixed asset accounting records be used in the hospital's preventive maintenance programs?

Chapter 14

Cash Management

In this chapter we will examine how to budget cash receipts, cash needs, sources of additional cash, and investments, and to maintain control of cash transactions. For our purposes, cash includes any medium of exchange that a bank will accept for deposit and credit to a depositor's account. For example, securities, checks, money orders, drafts, and money on deposit with banks are all acceptable for deposit at a bank and are included in our definition of cash.

EXTENT OF THE PROBLEM

In the previous chapter, we saw how cash was the key to the working capital management process. The hospital that holds too much cash is financially safe but is not maximizing the services it can provide to patients. The hospital that holds too little cash is maximizing the services it can provide patients in the short run but in the long run is jeopardizing its credit, its ability to provide employee satisfaction, and its ability to add services that require additional or updated equipment.

The more cash the hospital can effectively put to work, the greater the fulfillment of the hospital's goals, up to that point where the loss of liquidity prevents the taking of discounts or induces loss of suppliers. The scope of the problem is often difficult to grasp because many boards, administrators, and other executives believe that payroll is met directly out of net revenue and that new services are paid for directly out of profits. It is often difficult to realize that disbursements can be made only out of cash.

PATIENT REVENUE AS A SOURCE OF CASH

The most significant source of cash for any hospital is patient revenues. In the chapter on budgeting, we saw how to estimate patient revenue by month. In this section, we will estimate cash generated from patient revenue by month.

Deductions from Revenue

In completing the cash budget, we are interested only in expected net revenue. Contractual allowances, bad debts, free care, and other deductions from revenue must be subtracted from gross patient billings to arrive at expected cash receipts.

Medicare and Medicaid normally calculate in advance an interim billing rate. Many other cost-based third party payers also have interim billing rates. This interim rate is used to discount current billings. It should be remembered that this is a negotiated rate and that the hospital should strive to keep the interim rate high. The interim billing rate is used to convert current gross billings into expected cash receipts. For example, if the hospital's interim billing rate for Medicare is 85 percent, then for every $100 in gross billings to Medicare, the hospital can expect to receive $85. The difference of $15 is an interim contractual adjustment until the cost report is settled.

An estimated deduction from gross billings for free care, bad debt, employee discounts, or any other adjustment must be estimated. This deduction is normally computed as a percentage of gross billing.

After subtracting contractual adjustments and other deductions from gross billings, the estimated cash receipts from patient revenue are known. But calculating estimated cash receipts from patient revenue is only the first step. It does not indicate when the cash will be received, only how much will be received.

Collection Time Lag

The collection time lag is the key to converting expected patient revenue into expected cash receipts. This time lag should be calculated first separately for each major payer and then in the aggregate. The recent history of payments is the major factor in estimating average collection time lag.

Table 14–1 shows a worksheet used to analyze the collection time lag in Community Hospital.

An analysis similar to that in Table 14–1 should be made for Medicare, Medicaid, Blue Cross, and any other major identifiable payer. This kind of analysis can be very time-consuming because it means tracing every bill for two or three months through to final disposition. However, once the process is outlined, the task can be completed by temporary help.

After a worksheet has been completed for each major payer category, the results are summarized to arrive at an aggregate collection lag. The analysis could be completed in the aggregate. However, collection time lag by payer category also provides valuable information in that it allows a hospital to analyze cash budget variances more thoroughly.

Table 14–1 Community Hospital Worksheet To Analyze Collection Lag

January and February 19X0

Payer Type: Blue Cross

	Month of Billing		Total	
Month of Receipt	*January*	*February*	*Dollars*	*%*
Month billed	$ 31,050	$30,000	$ 61,050	28.7
First month	63,200	56,840	120,040	56.3
Second month	19,290	7,510	26,800	12.6
Third month	0	1,080	1,080	0.5
Fourth month	890	0	890	0.4
Fifth month	0	180	180	0.1
Sixth month	210	0	210	0.1
Still pending after six months	360	2,390	2,750	1.3
	$115,000	$98,000	$213,000	100.0

Assume the collection time lag is calculated to be 26.5 percent in the month of billing, 52.0 percent in the following month, 12.5 percent in the 3rd month, and 1.0 percent in the 4th through the 12th month following billing. Only an insignificant amount of expected cash from patient revenue is collected more than 12 months after billing. Now we subtract from projected gross patient billings by month an amount for contractual adjustments, bad debt, and free care to arrive at expected cash from patient revenue. By multiplying this result by the percentage estimated to be collected by month, we can arrive at an annual cash budget. Table 14–2 is a sample cash budget from patient revenue for Community Hospital.

Each hospital might set up its worksheets to calculate expected cash from patient billings in a different way. However, the principles should be similar to those in the methodology we have presented in this section.

OTHER SOURCES OF CASH

Other sources of cash may include cafeteria income, coffee shop income, vending machine and telephone rebates, tuition from nursing school, tuition from other programs, grants, payments for residency programs, transfers from endowments or other restricted funds, and donations. Almost all miscellaneous revenue is collected when earned. For purposes of cash budgeting, most hospitals include 1/12th of miscellaneous income in their forecast per month. Ex-

Table 14–2 Community Hospital Cash Budget from Patient Billings

For the Year Ended December 31, 19X0
in Thousands

Month Billed	Total	Jan.	Feb.	Mar.	Apr.	May	June	July	Aug.	Sept.	Oct.	Nov.	Dec.
Prior years	$ 1,255	$622	$175	$ 70	$ 74	$ 68	$ 72	$ 62	$ 39	$ 31	$ 22	$ 13	$ 7
January	881	233	457	110	9	9	9	9	9	9	9	9	9
February	850		228	447	107	8	9	8	9	8	9	8	9
March	841			228	447	107	8	9	8	9	8	9	8
April	816				223	438	105	8	8	9	8	8	9
May	797					220	432	104	8	8	8	8	8
June	807						225	442	106	8	9	9	9
July	807							228	447	107	8	8	8
August	811								231	453	109	9	9
September	774									223	438	105	8
October	745										217	426	102
November	613											207	406
December	188												188
Total	$10,185	$855	$860	$855	$860	$850	$860	$870	$865	$865	$845	$820	$780

ceptions to this would be such items as tuition, grants, transfers from restricted funds, and payments for residency programs. The timing of receipt of cash for these items can normally be accurately predicted by analyzing prior years.

Once cash receipts from nonpatient sources have been forecasted by month, the amounts are added to expected cash receipts from patient billings. The sum represents expected cash receipts from normal operations.

CASH DISBURSEMENTS

Cash disbursements include additions to working capital needs, payroll, payroll taxes and fringes, supplies and expense, and balance sheet disbursements. Because of the detail needed to estimate cash disbursements, a separate schedule should be prepared for each of these categories. The totals by month are then carried forward to the statement on the sources and uses of cash.

Working Capital Needs

In the previous chapter, we studied working capital management. It was demonstrated that working capital needs normally increase each year. Although this does not require a direct cash disbursement, it does require funds that would otherwise be available as cash. The effect on cash availability is the same as writing a check. For this reason, we should treat increased working capital needs as a cash disbursement.

The increased working capital needed for accounts receivable is greatest in the first three months of the year. This is because hospitals normally increase prices at the beginning of the fiscal year. We saw in studying collection time lag that most expected cash receipts from patient billings are collected in the first three months. After an analysis of the collection time lag, the increased working capital needed for accounts receivable can be accurately forecasted by month.

If the hospital needs any other major increase in working capital for a particular month, this should be calculated. Otherwise it can be assumed that increased working capital needs occur evenly throughout the year and that 1/12th is budgeted for each month.

Salaries and Wages

Payroll represents the most critical cash need for a hospital. Payroll cash is critical both because it is the largest cash need category and because the timing cannot be delayed for even a short period.

In an earlier chapter, the development of an expense budget for salaries and wages for payroll by month was illustrated. This expense budget is the starting point for the payroll cash budget.

The first calculation is the average expense per pay period by month. This should be calculated separately for each month of the fiscal year. The formula for the calculation is as follows:

$$\text{Average Expense Per Pay Period} = \frac{\text{Pay Period} \times \text{Budget Expense}}{\text{Days in Month}}$$

where:

Pay Period = number of actual days in the hospital's pay period

Budget Expense = actual budgeted salaries and wages expense for the applicable month taken from the hospital's expense budget worksheet

Days in Month = number of calendar days in the applicable month

For example, assume we are calculating the average expense per pay period for the month of January for a hospital that pays every two weeks. Assume the January salaries and wages expense budget for payroll is $1 million. The average expense per pay period in this example would be:

$$\text{Average Expense} = \frac{14 \times \$1,000,000}{31} = \$451,600$$

After we have calculated the average expense per pay period for every month, the next step is to determine the number of payrolls that the hospital will be required to meet in each month. If the hospital pays every two weeks, then normally ten of the months will have two payrolls and two of the months will have three payrolls. Approximately once every ten years, only nine months will have two pay periods and three months will have three pay periods.

Multiplying the average payroll expense by month times the number of expected payrolls required to be met in that month gives the approximate amount of cash.needed by month to meet base payroll. If vacations and paid holidays are included in the payroll salaries and wages expense budget, our cash required to meet base payroll will include these. If vacations and paid holidays are included in fringe benefits for payroll expense budgeting, our cash required to meet payroll salaries and wages would not include these amounts.

Federal withholding and Social Security taxes must be paid monthly. However, some state withholding taxes for deferred compensation or insurance are paid only quarterly. If the hospital has an employee withholding tax that is paid only quarterly, an adjustment will need to be made to the cash budget for salaries and wages to reflect this.

Payroll Taxes and Fringe Benefits

The next step is to calculate the cash required for payroll taxes and fringe benefits by month. This step will be more time-consuming than calculating cash requirements for salaries and wages.

An analysis must first be made to determine the payment due dates for each payroll tax and fringe benefit. These taxes and benefits include, but are not limited to, the employer portion of Social Security taxes, workmen's compensation, state unemployment insurance, federal unemployment insurance, contributions to pension funds, health insurance, life insurance, long-term disability insurance, bonuses if applicable, and vacation plus paid holidays if these are not included in salaries and wages expense.

For benefits that are determined on an annual basis by an actuary, the hospital may pay 1/12th each month. These could include pension fund contributions, workmen's compensation, life insurance, and long-term disability insurance. These amounts should be entered on the worksheet for cash required for payroll taxes and fringe benefits.

Most payroll taxes and fringe benefits are accrued as a percentage of gross salaries. For these benefits, the hospital must determine by month the percentage of gross salary expense represented by each payroll tax or fringe benefit. These percentages are then applied to the cash budget for salaries and wages per month, not to the expense budget for salaries and wages. This calculation produces a projected cash need generated by each month's salaries and wages.

The payment dates for each tax and benefit accrued must be determined as a percentage of gross salaries. Payments may be due monthly, quarterly, semiannually, annually, or on some other schedule. Once the hospital has calculated the cash required for taxes and benefits that accrue as a percentage of gross salaries and the payment due date for each applicable tax or fringe benefit is known, it becomes a simple matter to project cash requirements by month for these expenses.

Supplies and Expense

Supply and expense budgets by month have been forecasted in the hospital's expense budget. To convert the expense budget into a cash budget by month, a payment time lag must be computed. Just as collection time lag is the key to converting patient revenue to cash received from patient revenue, the payment time lag is the key to converting the monthly expense budget into the supplies and expense cash disbursements budget.

The first step in calculating the payment time lag is to isolate all noncash expense items and also any large expense items that have specific, erratic, or contractual terms. Noncash items include depreciation and amortization. These must be subtracted from the monthly expense projections. Significant specific, erratic, or contractual items include interest on long-term debt, insurance, utilities, some service contracts, large lease expenses, and any other items the hospital can identify. Care must be taken to subtract these items from the expense budget in exactly the same months in which they were budgeted.

To estimate the accounts payable time lag, the hospital divides the total nonsalary expense for a year by 365. This calculation is not adjusted for total nonsalary expense for specific, erratic, or contractual items as identified above. However, before making the calculation, depreciation and amortization must be substracted from annual nonsalary expense. This gives us the average daily nonsalary expense.

The average daily nonsalary expense is then divided into the accounts payable amount shown on the balance sheet. The result is the average number of days expense in accounts payable. This is a reasonable approximation of the hospital's payment time lag. The number of days is now rounded to the nearest month and used to convert the expense budget for supplies and expense into a cash budget. If the average payment lag is two months, we can assume for purposes of the cash budget that all of a month's expense will be paid in two months.

In practice, accounts payable management is more complicated than this. However, inconsistencies from month to month tend to offset each other. We have subtracted significant specific, erratic, or contractual items and also depreciation and amortization. Thus, the use of the average number of days expense in accounts payable to forecast cash needs for other supplies and expense is adequate for our purposes.

Balance Sheet Disbursements

The last category of cash disbursements to forecast is balance sheet disbursements. This represents cash required for those expenditures that are not currently expensed. It includes payments on both long-term and short-term debt. It also includes transfers to restricted funds, a depreciation fund, plant fund, construction fund, or self-insurance fund. The hospital will need to prepare a schedule that summarizes these cash needs by month.

Schedule of Cash Needs

Cash needs should be summarized on a schedule of cash disbursements. Table 14–3 is a typical cash disbursements schedule for Community Hospital.

Sources and Uses of Cash from Operations

Earlier in this chapter we discussed estimated cash receipts and estimated cash needs. Now the hospital is ready to prepare a schedule of the sources and

Table 14–3 Community Hospital Schedule of Cash Needs

For the Three Months Ended March 31, 19X0
in Thousands

Cash Need	Total	Jan.	Feb.	Mar.
Salaries and wages	$1,020	$350	$315	$ 355
Payroll taxes and fringe benefits	230	85	70	75
	1,250	435	385	430
Supplies and expense	675	230	210	235
Balance sheet disbursements	425	0	0	425
Working capital needs*	200	70	60	70
Total cash needs	$2,550	$735	$655	$1,160

* Not direct cash disbursements

uses of cash from operations. Table 14–4 shows a typical schedule of sources and uses of cash from operations for Community Hospital. In this table, a substantial cash surplus is forecasted for several months, and a cash deficiency is forecasted for other months. This is a typical situation not only in hospitals but in most other enterprises as well. The next steps are to plan temporary sources of cash for the deficiency months and temporary investments for the cash surplus months.

Level of Cash Needed

Before we can plan temporary sources of cash for the deficiency months and temporary investments for the cash surplus months, we must determine the level of cash needed by the hospital.

John Maynard Keynes identified three motives for holding cash: the transactions motive, the precautionary motive, and the speculative motive. The transactions motive refers to the need for the hospital to plan to have cash on hand to pay its obligations as they become due. For example, payment of wages creates a cash need on a day which is not matched by cash receipts for that day. Therefore, we start to build cash for several days in anticipation of payday. In like manner, accounts payable, petty cash disbursements, payments to contractors, and other transactions create predictable discrepancies between cash inflows (income) and cash outflows (disbursements).

The precautionary motive refers to the need for the hospital to maintain an identifiable amount of cash to meet unpredictable discrepancies between cash

Table 14–4 Community Hospital—Sources and Uses of Cash from Operations

For the Year Ended December 31, 19X0
in Thousands

	Total	Jan.	Feb.	Mar.	Apr.	May	June	July	Aug.	Sept.	Oct.	Nov.	Dec.
Beginning cash	$ 90	$ 90	$ 310	$ 615	$ 410	$ 625	$ 410	$ 730	$ 950	$ 745	$ (290)	$ (85)	$ (340)
Cash received													
Patient sources	10,185	855	860	855	860	850	860	870	865	865	845	820	780
Nonpatient sources	1,240	100	100	100	100	100	130	100	100	100	110	100	100
Total cash received	11,425	955	960	955	960	950	990	970	965	965	955	920	880
Cash available	11,515	1,045	1,270	1,570	1,370	1,575	1,400	1,700	1,915	1,710	655	835	540
Cash uses	11,665	735	655	1,160	745	1,165	670	750	1,170	2,000	750	1,175	690
Ending cash	$ (150)	$ 310	$ 615	$ 410	$ 625	$ 410	$ 730	$ 950	$ 745	$(290)	$ (85)	$ (340)	$ (150)

inflows and cash outflows. The amount of funds needed to satisfy precautionary motives depends upon the hospital's credit standing, the established temporary sources of cash, and the psychological profile of the chief financial officer. A hospital with a good credit standing and preestablished sources of temporary funds may not feel it necessary to hold any funds at all for unpredictable cash needs.

The speculative motive for holding cash is not applicable to a hospital. Once the targeted cash needs for the month are known, the hospital can compute the required borrowing necessary or the amount available for investment.

Assume that in our example the hospital does not see a need to hold cash for precautionary needs and has determined that, to satisfy the transactions motive, the average cash balance should be one percent of the month's expected cash disbursements. The amount of borrowing needed and the investment opportunity by month can be calculated as shown in Table 14–5.

The hospital is now ready to plan temporary investments and the sources of temporary cash needs.

TEMPORARY INVESTMENTS

A hospital must tailor its investment policy to include only relatively safe investments. For the sake of another percent interest yield, a hospital cannot

---

Table 14–5 Cash Borrowing/Investment Budget

For the Year Ending December 31, 19X0
in Thousands

	Budgeted Ending Cash	Borrowing Need	Investment Opportunity	One Percent Of Month's Cash Uses
January	$310		$236	$ 74
February	615		550	65
March	410		294	116
April	625		551	74
May	410		294	116
June	730		663	67
July	950		875	75
August	745		628	117
September	(290)	$490		200
October	(85)	160		75
November	(340)	458		118
December	(150)	219		69

risk the loss of principal that will be needed for operations in a few weeks or a few months. There are several kinds of relatively safe investments. Short-term investments can be managed either directly by the hospital or through the hospital's commercial bank or banks. The hospital should have an investment policy approved by its governing board and under that policy consider the following investments.

Treasury Securities

U.S. treasury securities constitute the largest and safest segment of the money markets. Treasury bills are auctioned weekly by the Treasury and normally carry maturities of 91 days to 182 days. The secondary market for these bills is very active. If funds are needed, the hospital can easily sell treasury bills before they mature.

The Treasury also offers treasury notes, which carry a maturity of from one to seven years. Because of the long maturities of these notes, a hospital would normally purchase and sell them only in the secondary markets. Other issues offered by the Treasury would not normally be used by hospitals.

Other Government Issues

The Federal Land Bank, the Federal Home Loan Bank, and other federal agencies are authorized to issue securities. These securities are not always guaranteed by the U.S. Government but are still highly regarded for short-term investment purposes.

State and local governments often issue securities, but the interest yield on them is usually low. Interest on these issues is exempt from taxes, but this is a quality that most hospitals cannot exploit.

Bankers Acceptances

Bank acceptances are drafts that are accepted by banks and used in the financing of foreign and domestic trade. With the growth in international trade, the volume of bank acceptances has grown rapidly. Acceptances generally have a maturity of less than 180 days, tend to have an effective interest rate slightly higher than treasury bills, and are generally of high quality. They are bought and sold in the over-the-counter market.

Commercial Paper

High-grade commercial paper is a promissory note issued by large, established corporations. Rates on commercial paper are higher than on treasury securities.

Commercial paper is sold on a discount basis and normally has maturities ranging from 30 to 270 days. Unlike treasury securities and bank acceptances, most commercial paper must be held to maturity. Arrangements may be made through dealers for the repurchase of commercial paper sold through them, but there is no established secondary market for these securities.

Repurchase Agreements

Repurchase agreements represent an investment opportunity that is widely used by hospitals. Government security dealers carry a large inventory of securities. These securities are sold to the hospital for short periods of time with an agreement by the dealer to repurchase them at a set price. Repurchase agreements are for short periods of time (such as over a weekend) and offer a yield that is slightly higher than treasury obligations. The repurchase agreement aids the dealer in carrying an inventory and, at the same time, offers the hospital a safe investment for temporary excess funds.

The above represents the major short-term investment opportunities for hospitals. Other investments used by commercial corporations, such as certificates of deposit, either have long maturities, no secondary market, or for some other reason do not usually fit the needs of hospitals. However, the investment needs of each hospital are unique. Investment opportunities not mentioned in this section should be carefully examined before assuming they are not appropriate. Risk, return, and marketability require ongoing analysis.

TEMPORARY SOURCES OF CASH

In this section, we will examine temporary sources of cash. Cash is needed on a temporary basis to meet budgeted cash deficiencies as well as to meet needs caused by unpredictable discrepancies between inflow and outflow of funds.

Delaying Disbursements

Postponing the payment of accounts payable is an expedient and inexpensive temporary source of funds as long as the hospital does not lose any purchase discounts. The only cost to the hospital (assuming there are no lost discounts) is the possible weakening of its credit standing with a particular supplier.

Disbursements of funds may also be delayed by paying large suppliers with a draft rather than by check. A draft is a negotiable instrument that orders the hospital's bank to pay a third party. The supplier presents the draft to the supplier's bank for payment. After several days, the draft is presented to the hospital's bank. The hospital has until the bank closes that day to inspect the draft and to deposit funds to cover it. Although the process seems cumbersome, it is relatively simple, and it provides a few additional days before the funds are required.

The hospital can also delay disbursements through the bank float. To accomplish this, the hospital calculates the amount of time it will take for a check mailed today to reach the bank. Normally, the hospital can depend on two or three days before a check mailed today is received and deposited by the supplier. Depending upon the location of the supplier, it can take up to two more days before the check is presented for payment at the hospital's bank. Therefore, a hospital can sometimes write a check and not have funds available to cover it for up to five working days. This source of funds should be used only occasionally and should be closely monitored because its use is discouraged by the bank.

Bank Credit

Many hospitals have established lines of credit with their banks. This is an agreement between the bank and the hospital that a loan up to a stated dollar limit will be granted as needed. Normally, these loans are unsecured and the interest rate is stated as a percentage above the bank's prime rate. By negotiating the loan terms ahead of time, the hospital and the bank both benefit. The line of credit commitment is normally renewed each year.

The hospital can also receive a single loan from a bank. The bank will consider each loan request on its individual merit. Even without a line-of-credit agreement, the hospital can borrow several times during the year.

It is becoming a common practice for banks to require borrowers to maintain minimum deposit balances that are related in some manner to the size of the line of credit or loan. Because these balances are intended to be a form of compensation to the bank, they are called compensating balances. Compensating balance requirements are quite sensitive to the amount of available funds at commercial banks. If money becomes tight, these requirements are rigidly enforced.

If the minimum compensating balance agreement is less than the hospital would normally keep in the bank, the requirement does not add to the effective interest rate. If the bank requires a higher balance than the hospital would normally maintain, however, there is an inputed interest expense. For example, assume the bank grants the hospital a $1,000,000 loan at eight percent interest. Assume also that the bank requires the hospital to maintain a compensating balance that is $50,000 higher than the hospital would normally keep. The true interest rate is calculated as follows.

$$\text{Effective Interest Rate} = \frac{\text{Quoted Interest Rate} \times \text{Amount Borrowed}}{\text{Amount Borrowed Minus Additional Balances}}$$

In our example, the effective interest rate is:

$$\frac{.08 \times \$1,000,000}{\$1,000,000 - \$50,000} = 8.42 \text{ percent}$$

By requiring the hospital to maintain additional funds on deposit, the bank has reduced the amount of available funds. The hospital is, in effect, paying interest on funds it cannot use. This technique increases the true interest rate on borrowed funds.

Daily Monitoring

We have discussed cash management on a monthly basis because the cash budget is normally prepared on a monthly basis. However, cash should be monitored on a daily basis. Cash needs and temporary excess cash situations are often of a short-term nature.

Methods of monitoring cash on a daily basis are developed by the chief financial officer to satisfy that executive's individual needs. The method may be informal, or it may be as formalized as the monthly budget. However, the method should be formal enough to at least consider such items as timing of payroll disbursements, timing of payroll withholding deposits and payroll taxes, and possible weekly receipt of checks from third party payers (i.e., Blue Cross, Medicare). Exhibit 14–1 shows a daily cash monitoring form. The form shows

Exhibit 14–1 Community Hospital Daily Cash Sheet

January, 19XX							
Cash Received				*Cash Disbursed*			
Average Daily: Budgeted	*Average Daily: Actual*	*Days Receipts*		*Days Checks*	*Average Daily: Actual*	*Average Daily: Budgeted*	
			Date				

Receipt Notes:
1. Blue Cross checks of $300,000 (approx.) received Tuesday each week
2. Medicare PIP check of $750,000 received Jan. 15 and 30

Disbursement Notes:
1. Payroll $500,000 (approx.) due on Jan. 13 and 27
2. Payroll of $1,000,000 (approx.) will be paid approximately Jan. 20
3. Transfer to plant fund of $130,000 on Jan. 30

daily budgeted amounts, month-to-date average daily receipts and disbursements, and daily activity. In addition, there is a section at the bottom to write short reminders of significant receipts or disbursements. These notes are completed at the beginning of the month when the form is prepared.

The actual form used by individual hospitals may vary substantially from this example. However, it should be cautioned that if the daily cash form has too much information, it may exceed the ability of the administrative staff to absorb. Any report that is prepared daily must be kept short and simple. Complicated or extensive information presented on a daily basis will be ignored by most busy administrators.

SUMMARY

Patient revenue represents the most significant source of hospital cash. To estimate cash receipts from patient revenues, we subtract interim rate adjustments, contractual adjustments, bad debt, discounts, and free care from expected gross patient revenue. The largest deductions will normally be for interim rate adjustments. After subtracting allowances and contractual adjustments from revenue, we have expected cash receipts from patients. This projects how much will be received, but it does not project when it will be received. After calculating a collection time lag, we can project cash receipts from patients by month. Nonpatient sources of cash include sources such as the cafeteria, coffee shop, vending machines, telephone rebates, tuition, residency program payments, donations, and transfers from other funds.

Cash disbursements include additions to working capital, payroll, payroll taxes and fringes, supplies, other expenses, and balance sheet disbursements. Although working capital needs do not require a direct cash disbursement, they do require funds that would otherwise be available as cash. In addition to cash requirements, the hospital must plan to hold enough cash to satisfy the precautionary motives of the board and administration.

The difference between projected cash needs and projected cash receipts represents either a temporary investment opportunity or a temporary cash need. The most common temporary investments include treasury securities, other government issues, bankers acceptances, commercial paper, and repurchase agreements. Sources of cash to fill temporary needs include the delaying of disbursements, line-of-credit arrangements, and loans.

In addition to developing a schedule of monthly sources and use of cash, it is important to monitor cash within the month on a daily basis. The minimum daily cash monitoring needs are payroll disbursements, payroll withholding and tax deposits, and receipt of large checks from third party payers.

DISCUSSION QUESTIONS

1. Discuss what is wrong with a hospital holding too much cash or too little cash.
2. What is meant by the term *third party interim rate?*
3. How is the collection time lag used to convert expected cash receipts from patients into a cash receipts forecast?
4. Why is the cash budget for salaries, wages, and fringe benefits different from the expense budget for salaries, wages, and fringe benefits?
5. Discuss some items that should be considered in determining the level of cash needed.
6. Discuss several temporary investment opportunities available to hospitals.
7. Discuss several temporary sources of cash available to hospitals.

Chapter 15

Taxation

In this chapter we will examine tax exempt status, employee retirement income, and other tax matters. The principles covered will be broad and do not represent an exhaustive coverage of the subject. We will, however, attempt to give the reader a good understanding of the complex problems of taxation, even for a tax-exempt hospital.

TAX-EXEMPT ORGANIZATIONS

Most American hospitals are tax exempt and, therefore, not required to pay taxes on related business income. This exemption is either because the hospital is part of a local, state, or federal political subdivision or because the hospital has applied for and been granted a tax-exempt status by the Internal Revenue Service.

501 (C) (3) Organizations

Most hospitals are exempt from income tax under Internal Revenue Code Section 501 (C) (3). This section reads in part that the following may gain tax-exempt status:

> [A] corporation and any community chest, fund, or foundation organized and operated exclusively for religious, charitable, scientific testing for public safety, literary or educational purposes, or to foster national or international amateur sports competition or for the prevention of cruelty to children or animals, no part of the net earnings of which inures to the benefit of any private shareholder or individual, no substantial part of the activities of which is carrying on propaganda,

or otherwise attempting to influence legislation and which does not attempt to participate or intervene in any political campaign.

To receive exemption under Section 501 (C) (3), the hospital must file a Form 1023. This form is available from any Internal Revenue Service (IRS) office. Part of the form asks for a description of the operations of the business. Income that is earned within the scope of these operations is not taxed. However, if the hospital has income from the operation of a business not related to the purpose stated in the exemption, it will be required to pay income taxes on this nonrelated income. This is taxed at the corporate tax rates in effect at the time, but the first $1,000 of nonrelated income in any calendar year is exempt from tax.

It is important that the hospital protect its tax-exempt status. The IRS can and often does revoke the exempt status of hospitals and other organizations. Exempt status is revoked when the hospital participates in partisan political activity or performs actions in which the tax-exempt status is used to benefit a private individual. The kinds of actions that may jeopardize the exempt status are best illustrated by the following examples.

The use of hospital funds to influence legislation will jeopardize the exempt status if the funds can be interpreted as being substantial in relation to the hospital's total expenditures. All hospitals contribute to some lobbying. A significant part of the dues to the American Hospital Association is used for lobbying. The key point is to keep lobbying and other expenditures to influence legislation less than substantial in relation to the hospital's total expenditures.

Hospitals can lose exempt status by engaging in activities that benefit a private individual or organization. The following practices have resulted in revocation of a hospital's tax-exempt status: unduly restricting use of the hospital's facilities to a certain group of physicians; paying salaries or extending service, supply, or other payments to an individual or organization in excess of the going market price; making loans without adequate security or without provision for a reasonable interest rate; and not dealing at "arms length" in contract negotiations.

In addition to being required to pay taxes on income, there are several other problems that may arise if a hospital's tax-exempt status is lost. The first problem is that donations to the hospital will no longer qualify as charitable deductions on the donors' tax returns. Another problem relates to the disposition of assets. In order to obtain tax-exempt status, the hospital charter had to include a clause stating that, when the corporation ceases to exist, the assets will be distributed to tax-exempt organizations. This becomes a problem because a hospital that has lost its exempt status ceases to qualify, and continual use of its assets may not be automatic. These are some of the problems that may arise if the hospital loses its tax exemption. The revocation can be retroactive. In reality, however, exempt status is seldom revoked retroactively.

Information Returns

Most tax-exempt hospitals are required to file an annual return with the IRS that records income, receipts, contributions, deductions from income, expenses, and other information. This information is reported on Form 990, *Return of Organization Exempt from Income Tax.* Failure to file this return by the due date will subject the hospital to a penalty.

Exempt income includes income from all activities that are related to the hospital's purpose. Generally, dividends, interest, annuities, and royalties are considered related business income and are not taxed. The rules and regulations covering exempt income are very difficult to interpret, and the hospital should seek professional advice if there is any doubt.

Unrelated Business Income

If the hospital engages in business activities that are not related to its exempt purpose, it must file a Schedule 990T. This schedule reports the unrelated business income, expenses, and net profit. An unrelated business is a venture that does not easily fit into the scope of activities for which the hospital was granted tax-exempt status. For example, if the hospital purchased an apartment house and rented the units, tax would have to be paid on the rental income. If it were not for this provision, General Motors, Ford, and other industrial giants could purchase or build a small tax-exempt hospital, transfer all of its assets to the hospital, and not pay tax on its millions in profits. If an entity is exempt because it is a hospital, it is only fair to tax profits that are not hospital-related.

There are several types of hospitals that may be exempt from paying taxes on unrelated business income. These include hospitals that are an instrumentality of a government or political subdivision and church-owned hospitals under certain circumstances.

Unrelated business income must be regularly carried on to be taxable, and the first $1,000 per hospital is specifically exempt. In addition, there are many complex rules that can be used to exclude income from taxation. Most hospitals need professional outside assistance to properly file and minimize income taxes on their Form 990T.

Hospitals have been searching for alternative sources to expand their revenue base. This trend will continue with increasing vigor as government programs, public pressure, and other influences grow. A whole new concept of tax planning is evolving in the American hospital industry.

EMPLOYEE RETIREMENT INCOME

Most hospitals have pension plans for employees. The enforcement of government regulations covering these plans is assigned to the IRS, the Department of Labor, and the Pension Benefit Guaranty Corporation.

General Provisions

Hospital employee pension funds may provide disability benefits, retirement benefits, deferred income plans, and annuity plans. Contributions are normally paid by the hospital, but in some cases the contributions are made jointly by the hospital and the employees.

There are four distinct persons or entities defined in a pension plan. These are the plan administrator, the plan sponsor, the plan participant, and a beneficiary. The plan administrator is either the hospital entity itself or a person specifically identified by the terms of the plan. The plan sponsor is normally either the hospital or a hospital association acting for several hospitals. The plan participant is any employee or former employee who is or may become eligible to receive benefits. A beneficiary is a person other than the employee who is designated to receive benefits under the plan.

An annual report on all pension plans must be filed with the Department of Labor within 210 days after the end of the plan year. Other reports that may be required to be filed with the Department of Labor include underlying documents on request, a plan description and summary of plan description four months after the plan is subject to reporting requirements, changes in plan description two months after a change or modification occurs, and an updated plan description when requested but not more frequently than once every five years.

There are also reports that must be filed with the Pension Benefit Guaranty Corporation for plans covered by termination insurance. The IRS requires an annual registration statement, notification of change in status for plans subject to vesting standards, annual returns, and an actuarial report for the first year of funding and every third year thereafter. A critical due date list should be established to make sure that all required reports are filed when due.

There are also certain information reports that must be given to participants and beneficiaries. These include a summary annual report of the plan, an updated plan description every ten years if unchanged and every five years if changed, a summary of changes in the plan, and summary plan descriptions. Written explanations are required to be sent to any participant or beneficiary whose claims are denied.

Failure to comply with any disclosure or reporting requirements may subject the hospital to a fine of up to $100,000. Other penalties can be levied for small specific incidences involving communications between beneficiaries and the plan.

Fiduciary Provisions

Fiduciary provisions under the law prohibit certain transactions, pinpoint control and responsibility for the administration of funds, and mandate other requirements. These provisions are administered by the Department of Labor.

Retirement income plans cannot engage in transactions that directly or indirectly benefit parties who have an interest in the plan. This includes plan administrators, employees of a plan, persons performing services to the plan, the employer of covered employees, and others. Exceptions to prohibited transactions include loans available to all participants or beneficiaries on a nondiscriminatory basis and other arms-length transactions defined in the law.

Because of the complex and changing provisions of the law, most hospitals do not administer their own employee pension plans. The plans are rather administered by the trust department of a bank, by insurance companies, by consultants, or by others.

Other Tax Matters

For-profit hospitals must annually file a corporate, partnership, or self-employment income tax return. The form required depends upon the type of hospital ownership. Principles of taxation are beyond the scope of this book. It should be noted, however, that approximately ten percent of American hospitals are for-profit. It cannot be assumed that nonprofit status is always the most beneficial. With certain employment tax credits, investment credits, depreciation methods, and other credits, the amount of income tax paid can be kept to a minimum. Moreover, for-profit hospitals receive more reimbursement on third-party cost reports. Medicare and Medicaid allow a reasonable return on equity invested as an addition to costs when filing the cost reports. It may be beneficial for a nonprofit hospital to study the advantages of becoming taxable. The most beneficial time to elect this change in status would be immediately after a major expansion has been financed. At this point in a hospital's history, assets and liabilities are relatively equal, and the book value of assets being converted is relatively small.

Hospitals must closely monitor sales and real estate tax provisions. These state and local taxes are complex and vary from one locality to another. All hospitals collect and pay sales taxes on gift shop sales. Many collect and pay sales taxes on cafeteria sales, coffee shop sales, take-home drugs, and other special sales. Depending upon the locality, the hospital may owe real estate tax on rental property, parking garages, and auxiliary enterprises. The hospital should never begin paying any of these taxes until it is clearly necessary. Taxing authorities are often overly ambitious to discover new sources of income. The hospital can set an undesirable precedent by paying a new tax before it has thoroughly researched the provisions of the tax law. At the same time, the hospital must be careful to avoid paying interest and penalties on past-due taxes. Professional advice should be obtained whenever there is a question that cannot be adequately resolved by hospital personnel.

Audits are performed on hospitals by the IRS, state sales tax agencies, the Department of Labor, state and local payroll income tax agencies, and others. It is important to plan for and manage carefully any tax examination. A hospital employee should be designated to coordinate each tax audit. This employee should maintain a log of all records forwarded to and returned from the auditors. The employee should insist upon being present when any other hospital employees are interviewed by the auditors and should keep notes on what is asked, what answers are given, and impressions of the audit. These records and logs should be kept at least until the results of the audit and any audit adjustments are finalized.

SUMMARY

Most American hospitals are tax exempt under Internal Revenue Code Section 501(C) (3). Others are tax exempt because they are a subdivision of a local, state, or federal government. Exemption from taxes does not mean exemption from filing reports or from management of tax matters. An annual information return must be filed and income taxes paid on income that is not within the scope of the exemption certificate. Numerous reports are required on employee pension plans. Sales taxes, real estate taxes, and other taxes are paid by hospitals. It is important to minimize taxes to all government agencies while protecting the hospital from penalties and interest on past-due taxes.

Tax-exempt status should not be taken for granted. The IRS has revoked the exempt status of hospitals that participate in influencing legislation, perform actions that benefit a private individual, or indulge in other proscribed activities. It should also be noted that a tax-exempt status may not always be the most beneficial status for a hospital. There are many advantages that are enjoyed only by for-profit hospitals.

Audits are regularly performed on hospitals by the IRS, state sales tax agencies, the Department of Labor, state and local payroll income tax agencies, and by other agencies. The hospital should assign to a specific employee the responsibility for monitoring all audits. This employee should keep a record of items examined by the auditors, employees questioned, and other audit activities. Only by carefully managing a tax audit can the hospital minimize its potential liability.

DISCUSSION QUESTIONS

1. Explain some of the conditions that must be met to become a tax-exempt organization.
2. What is unrelated business income? Why should the hospital be required to pay taxes on this income?
3. List several examples of ways in which a hospital could lose its tax-exempt status.
4. List some of the reports that must be filed on employee pension plans and their frequency.
5. What are some of the fiduciary provisions required under the law pertaining to employee pension plans?
6. What considerations should guide the hospital's position in collecting and paying taxes on sales, real estate, and other similar assessments?

Chapter 16

Hospital Feasibility Studies

Occasionally a hospital will undertake a major feasibility study to determine debt capacity, to prepare for a bond issue, or in conjunction with a long-term plan. Although these studies can be done internally, they are normally done by a consulting firm or by a certified public accounting firm.

In this chapter, we will examine the components of a hospital feasibility study. Not all feasibility studies will include all of the steps enumerated. Rather our discussion will serve as a guide in negotiating a feasibility study with an outside firm, as an outline for a hospital that wishes to perform such a study with its own staff, or as a guide for a hospital executive who needs a clear understanding of what is included in a hospital feasibility study.

CHOOSING THE STUDY TEAM

In this section, we will outline several considerations in choosing an outside firm for a feasibility study or in deciding to perform such a study with the hospital's staff.

Certified Public Accountants

In choosing a certified public accounting firm, the hospital must first evaluate its own needs. If a public debt issue is contemplated, a national certified public accounting firm that has performed many hospital studies is best. The bond-rating agencies and the investing public look favorably upon studies performed by national certified public accounting firms. Thus, the hospital's bonds or other debt instruments will attract a broader market. The hospital may even be able to obtain a lower interest rate.

A large firm that has conducted many hospital studies will have a firm set of standards that must be met. Nevertheless, the hospital must rely on the judgment

259

of the individuals who perform the study. This is a negotiable point, and the hospital should insist upon approving the resumes of the personnel who will be involved in its study. The hospital should also attempt to negotiate the amount of involvement of the firm's national health care consultants. Feasibility studies performed by the local office of a large, reputable certified public accounting firm may be of marginal quality.

The large national firms have a set of standards that they use to decide whether or not to accept the hospital as a client. For a full-scope study, they will insist on appropriate planning agency approval, on firm construction bids, or a documented guaranteed maximum price for any construction; and they stipulate certain hospital characteristics that must exist. For example, if the hospital is not at least 75 percent third party reimbursed, several large firms will not perform a feasibility study. This is because self-pay patients' payment and usage patterns cannot be accurately predicted in our economic system. Third party reimbursement is not affected significantly by economic conditions.

If the hospital contemplates a public debt offering, the firm will do an in-depth analysis of the hospital before contracting to perform a feasibility study. In addition, the firm will insist upon a carefully designed set of review procedures for which the hospital will be billed. Its proposal will delineate the work that the firm will perform and will clearly state that a change in scope may result in additional billings. The hospital will be required to submit a client's letter of representations stating that the assumptions and representations are agreed to by the hospital.

Consultants

Many consulting firms also perform feasibility studies. Depending upon the size of the firm and its experience with health care financial feasibility studies, a consulting firm may or may not perform a credible study. Many consulting firms do not have the review standards and the scope of procedures that certified public accounting firms enjoy.

If the hospital contemplates a public debt offering, only the large national consulting firms should be considered. This will ensure the marketability and rating of the issue. If the hospital is contemplating a private placement of its debt, any firm with an excellent reputation can be used. As in contracting with a certified public accounting firm, the consultants who will be assigned to the study, billable expenses, involvement of principals, and other matters related to the study are all negotiable. If the hospital is very aggressive in negotiating, the result will be a better study at the same or at lower costs than if extensive negotiations are not undertaken.

In-House Staff

A hospital that is planning a feasibility study can have outside consultants perform the entire study, can perform the entire study with existing hospital personnel, or can contract with a consultant to direct the study with some of the work completed by hospital personnel. A study completed entirely by outside consultants is expensive, will not be well-tailored to the needs of the institution, and offers no opportunity for staff development. However, it would be the easiest way for the hospital to complete the study. On the other hand, doing a feasibility study entirely with existing staff is difficult, has the greatest propensity for error, and generally will have the lowest credibility with the governing board. It is, however, inexpensive and offers the greatest opportunity for staff development.

Most hospital feasibility studies are performed by a consulting firm or by outside certified public accountants with some of the work performed by the hospital staff. It is to the hospital's advantage to do as much of the work as possible. The name of the outside firm, its reliance on quality standards, and the marketability of the study are the same whether the study is performed entirely by the outside consultants or with heavy hospital involvement. Moreover, completing portions of the study with the existing staff enables the hospital to develop its personnel, significantly reduces the consulting fees, and results in a study that will more closely meet the hospital's needs.

FORECASTING DEMAND

The next phase of any feasibility study involves the forecasting of demand for the hospital's services. In this section, we will present a comprehensive approach to forecasting demand for services. This would apply to a typical forecast for a public bond issue.

Preparing for the Forecast

To prepare for a feasibility analysis, the hospital should gather and analyze the information to be used. There are three kinds of studies that require demand forecasts. They are studies for debt capacity determination, studies for bond offerings, and long-range planning studies. The information needs are the same for all three. The information concerning the hospital's market area should include the names, addresses, administrators, and expansion plans of any hospitals, laboratories, clinics, or other health care providers in the service area. Relevant demographic studies by universities, health planning agencies, governments, or other researchers should be collected. If more than one study on the age, population density, economic prospects, and other characteristics of the people in the service area has been completed, the hospital should obtain all of these and compare them. The one that appears to be the most accurate should be used to forecast population and economic trends. If these studies have been used to forecast bed needs or other health care delivery needs, their forecasts should be studied.

Information on the hospital to be gathered will include copies of certificates of need and other planning agency applications and approvals, as well as schematic drawings, blueprints, reports, and other data used in planning expansion projects. A list of the members of the governing board and key committee members, organization charts for the present as well as the future, and names of department heads should be gathered. If the hospital has had a previous feasibility study, a copy of it should be obtained, even if it was performed many years ago. Copies should also be obtained of any official statements, bond prospectuses, or loan agreements.

The most important information to be gathered pertains to the hospital's medical staff. Information on the age, specialty, years in the community, certifications and board eligibility, and affiliations with other hospitals should be obtained for all staff physicians.

Defining the Service Area

All feasibility studies are based on assumptions about the supply and demand of patient care. The supply depends largely on the medical staff. Demand depends on the characteristics of the population. Both start with a definition of the service area.

Demand analysis begins with a patient-origin study. For every major type of admission, the address of the patient is examined. This will require separate analyses of inpatient admissions, the emergency room, and the outpatient clinic. After this is completed, it is often helpful to identify inpatient admissions by type of service. If the hospital is in a heavily populated urban area, a patient-origin study by zip code may be sufficient. For specialty hospitals, for rural hospitals, and for hospitals in small communities, the study will have to define areas on a map and classify patients according to these defined areas. Often these areas or communities are not defined until the accountant or consultant begins to study a small patient-origin sample.

The patient-origin studies should, if possible, cover periods of time from different quarters of the year. Although a month from each quarter would be ideal, this may be too voluminous to work with. A week from each of four quarters is a better statistical sample than four weeks from one quarter.

The patient-origin study defines the primary and the secondary geographic areas from which the hospital obtains its patients. The sample should include inpatients, emergency room patients, and clinic patients. Any unusual service area patterns should be investigated. For example, the hospital may be a regional referral center for a particular type of service, the emergency room patients may come predominantly from a small section of the city, or clinic patients may come from another section of the city. Once the patient service areas are defined, the conclusions should be explained to the chief executive of the hospital and, where appropriate, to the local health systems agency. Any changes suggested by the chief executive or outside agency should be incorporated into the study. Once the service areas are defined, demographic and economic factors of these areas should be studied.

In addition to identifying the demand service area, it is important to identify the supply service area for health care. The supply includes physicians as well as hospitals and clinics. The first step in the identification of the supply service level is to identify the location of the offices of the medical staff, of clinics, and of other hospitals in the area. The second step is to perform a patient-origin study that identifies the name and location of the physicians for inpatients and, if appropriate, for emergency room and clinic patients. Although this is a separate study from the demand patient-origin study, the collection of the data is performed simultaneously on the same patient admissions. For primary care physicians, the patients' residences and doctors' offices will normally be in the same geographic area. For specialists, this may not be the case.

The hospital should then consider any projected revisions or additions contemplated by competing hospitals, changes in the locations of doctors' offices, expected additions to the medical staff, and any topographical factors that may limit ease of access. The hospital should now be prepared to draw preliminary conclusions relative to a need for new specialties, growth in services, and other factors.

Physician Interviews

As the above information is being collected, the accountant or consultant will start physician interviews. The size and makeup of the medical staff will significantly affect the extent to which present and future facilities will be utilized. The physician interviews are often the most important part of the demand study.

In a large hospital, a comprehensive questionnaire is sent to all members of the medical staff. When these questionnaires are returned, follow-up interviews are conducted with an adequate sample of the physicians to determine that the responses indicated on the questionnaire are consistent with attitudes and opinions solicited in direct conversation. For a small hospital, and if time permits in a larger hospital, all of the staff physicians are interviewed.

To ensure consistency in interviewing and to ensure that all pertinent issues are fully covered, an interview guide should be used. The interview guide will be unique to the particular hospital. A sample interview guide for Community Hospital is shown in Exhibit 16–1. After conducting the physician interviews, the analyst should summarize the data collected and prepare a report on the conclusions and findings.

Interviews with Area Officials

In addition to conducting physician interviews, the analyst will talk to as many of the area health care officials as possible. Although these interviews are not as vital as the physician interviews, they provide an important new perspective to the forecast. Interviews should be held with major third party payers, hospital administrators, state and local health planning agencies, selected industrial executives, and financial lending executives.

Blue Cross, Medicare intermediary, and other major third party payers should be interviewed to determine what changes are contemplated in third party contracts or reimbursement principles. These agencies should also be asked to compare the hospital with other provider expansion programs and to indicate what changes are most likely in length of stay, admissions per thousand of population, and in other matters. The impact of future legislation should also be discussed with major third party payers. Any changes in admissions screening or utilization review that may be forthcoming should be discussed and their potential impact on the hospital's patient days determined.

If the analyst is given an interview by a hospital administrator in the area, the questions should begin with general information about the health care delivery in the area and end with specific questions about the administrator's own hospital. Some administrators will not discuss particular points relating to their hospitals but will reply to questions about the community. Information should be solicited about health maintenance organizations, commercial clinical services such as radiology or laboratory, proposed shared services, and other factors that could affect the hospital demand for health care services. Other matters that could be discussed include prospective rate changes, expansion plans that include new services or new construction, present or proposed relationships with other providers regarding diagnostic services, shared services or other understandings, and current utilization of inpatients and emergency room visits.

Health planning agencies should be asked about their projected bed needs and projected availability of physicians and other health care personnel. They should also be asked to supply information on certificate-of-need applications from other providers. The planning agency should be told about the hospital's expansion plans, and its verbal approval of the project should be sought. It is important to leave the planning agency with some supportive data and a very positive attitude in these initial stages.

Exhibit 16–1 Community Hospital—Physician Interview Guide

Interview Questions

1. In what ways are health care trends in this area different from national trends?
2. How are existing facilities meeting the need for health care delivery? What additional facilities are needed?
3. What facility expansions by hospitals are you aware of in this area? By physicians' groups? By clinics?
4. What can the hospital do to attract more physicians?
5. What significant changes do you feel will occur in this area's population? In its economy?
6. What is the hospital's strongest medical specialty? What is its weakest medical specialty?
7. How would you rank this hospital with other hospitals in the local area? In the region?
8. Explain the hospital's expansion plans and ask each physician:
   a. How many patients per month or per year do you expect to admit?
   b. What do you anticipate will be the average length of stay for your patients? For all patients?
   c. What do you anticipate your use of ancillary services will be as compared to present usage?
   d. How will physicians in general change their usage of ancillary services?
9. What do you think about the hospital's services, such as obstetrics, pediatrics, and surgery? Which of these should be eliminated and why? Which should be expanded and why?
10. How do your patients use the emergency room services? The clinics? The referred outpatient services?
11. What do you see changing in any of the areas asked about in the above ten questions?
12. What additions to or deletions from the current medical staff do you foresee?
13. What changes are beginning to take place in physician referral patterns at the hospital? What changes are most likely to take place in the future?
14. What trends do you see in health care for this area? What new health care programs do you see a need for in this area?
15. Do you support the hospital's proposed expansion plans? Why?

Industrial executives should be asked about planned changes in the work force. If a plant expansion is being considered that will bring additional families into the area, this should be noted. On the other hand, if a plant closing is being planned that will reduce the employment of the community, that is equally important. An industrial executive may know of a plant closing or a plant expansion being considered by another company that he cannot discuss definitively. However, the analyst should try to get a general feeling for changes in the work force even if definitive information is not available. The industrial executive can also be asked about proposed changes in employee health care benefit plans and any new eligibility requirements that may go into effect.

Financial lending executives should be asked to comment on future economic trends that they foresee on a national level as well as in the community being served by the hospital. The hospital's general credit standing and ability to support new debt should be discussed. Bankers, savings and loan officials, and other financial executives can also be asked about demographic studies they have prepared. Banks will have prepared population growth estimates in planning locations for new branches. Savings and loan companies watch new construction, buying and selling trends in real estate, and other factors that may have an effect upon the economy of the primary and secondary service areas.

Physicians, hospital administrators, bankers, industrial leaders, and others will of course not respond to all questions asked, nor will they share all of the information available to them. The consultant or accountant performing interviews should therefore be prepared for some rejections, evasive answers, and vague opinionated responses. In total, however, the interviews should prove to be worthwhile and will add an important dimension to the planning process.

Making the Estimate

The first part of the actual estimate is a mathematical exercise. Hospital usage projections by type of service per one thousand of population are available. The analyst should choose two or three different such projections and then make an informed choice as to what the hospital usage will be. Standards of health care need can be calculated using average usage rates in comparable communities in the state or nation, national urban area statistics, current and projected use rate formulas by medical specialty, state and local health planning agency formulas, and federal guidelines. By multiplying projected population in the service area by projected usage, the analyst can determine a projected hospital usage for the community.

The estimated usage should be adjusted for seasonal patterns in the community, such as an influx of college students or summer tourists. The statistics may also be adjusted for unusual characteristics in the population of the service area, such as age distribution, predominant occupations, and other factors. These adjusted usage estimates are then compared to the total facilities available. The hospital's market share is estimated, and statistics are developed for the hospital by year.

Once estimates of patient days have been made, they should be examined for reasonableness. The consultant or accountant should compare projected patient days and other statistics to impressions learned from:

- interviews with hospital officials

- interviews with industrial leaders

- interviews with financial executives

- trends developed from historical data.

After the projections have been adjusted for any apparent errors due to one or more of the above four comparisons, the statistical findings should be compared with the physicians' attitudes toward growth. All major discrepancies between the physicians' expectations and growth measured by statistical means must be investigated and fully explained before relying on the figures.

After patient days, emergency room visits, and clinic visits have been projected, utilization statistics should be forecasted for ancillary departments. Using demographic information from the primary and secondary service areas as well as standard ancillary usage projections by type of patient, the analyst can make a preliminary projection of ancillary usage. This projection is then compared to the physicians' expectations and any major discrepancies are resolved.

The next step in a feasibility study is to develop a set of proforma financial statements by year. This phase involves an assumption process, the preparation of projected financial statements, and a determination of the end use of the results.

THE ASSUMPTION PROCESS

Expense Assumptions

Before financial statements are prepared, the hospital will need to make many assumptions that will affect its financial statements. The number and specific nature of the assumptions will depend on the particular hospital, the computer simulation model to be used, and the judgment of the consultant or accountant. If a computer simulation model will not be used, the assumption process is especially critical, because changes in an assumption after the financial statements are prepared is a time-consuming and expensive process.

Most forecasting models convert outpatient occasions of service into equivalent patient days. Inpatient days and equivalent outpatient days are added together to get adjusted patient days. To convert the outpatient occasions to inpatient day equivalents, it is necessary to forecast an appropriate outpatient deflator. Intensity of service is defined as the amount of personnel, supplies, equipment, and other direct costs required to satisfy an average patient's need. The deflator converts the intensity of outpatient occasions of service to equivalent inpatient days so that all statistics are reduced to a common denominator. This is accomplished through the following four formulas:

1. Average Gross Outpatient Revenue Yield $= \dfrac{\text{Outpatient Charges}}{\text{Outpatient Occasions of Service}}$

2. Average Gross Inpatient Revenue Yield $= \dfrac{\text{Inpatient Charges}}{\text{Inpatient Days}}$

3. Outpatient Deflator $= \dfrac{\text{Average Outpatient Revenue Yield}}{\text{Average Inpatient Revenue Yield}}$

4. Adjusted Patient Days $= \text{Inpatient Days} + \left[\text{Outpatient Occasions} \times \text{Outpatient Deflator} \right]$

Historic national trends in the outpatient deflator by year are published by the American Hospital Association. By using the particular hospital's experience and national trends, the hospital's deflator can be estimated and total adjusted patient days computed for the forecast period.

The next important assumption used in forecasting models is productivity as measured by paid hours per adjusted patient day. Historically, there has been a decrease in hospital productivity over time due to such variables as increased technology, increased inpatient acuity levels, and employment conditions. The formula for productivity is:

$$\text{Productivity} = \dfrac{\text{Total Paid Hours}}{\text{Adjusted Patient Days}}$$

Comparative paid hours per adjusted patient day is available by bed size as well as by region. Using comparative data and hospital historical data, productivity is forecast throughout the study period.

Average hourly pay is used to project salary expense per full-item equivalent employee. The average pay increase experienced each year is determined by management judgment, the prevailing job market, inflation, the mix of high paid to low paid personnel, and the availability of necessary skills. The formula is:

$$\frac{\text{Total Projected Salary Expense}}{\text{Total Projected Paid Hours}} = \text{Average Hourly Pay Rate}$$

Comparative national data are available by bed size. Regional salary trends are normally available from several sources. These comparative data are used to project hourly pay rate increases.

Fringe benefits must be projected as a percentage of total gross salaries. Pension plan contributions, Social Security, health insurance, group life insurance, and other fringe benefits as a percent of total salary have been and should continue to increase each year. This is due to various government mandates as well as trends in personnel management to provide more benefits. The formula to compute this assumption, based on the hospital's trend compared with national trends, is:

$$\frac{\text{Total Employee Benefit Expense}}{\text{Total Salary Expense}} = \begin{array}{c}\text{Benefits As a Percent}\\ \text{of Gross Salaries}\end{array}$$

Professional fees per adjusted patient day include only those fees that the hospital bills on behalf of the physician. Any professional fee for which the physician bills directly is excluded from both hospital revenue and expense data. The annual percentage increase in professional fees per adjusted patient day should approximate the percentage increase in local salaries. If the hospital acts only as an intermediary in collecting professional fees, the impact of this assumption will not be great, because changes in the amount of fees collected will be offset by changes in the amount of fees paid. If a hospital has physicians on a fixed salary, however, this assumption becomes more critical.

Administrative and general expenses per licensed bed include all nonsalary expenses for employee health, personnel, data processing, admitting, purchasing, accounting, business office, and administration. Licensed beds are used rather than projected beds in use because administrative expenses are affected more by the size of the institution than by the number of beds open in any given year. This expense will normally increase at a rate consistent with the nation's overall Consumer Price Index.

Utilities per thousand of building gross square feet are normally forecast separately in a long-range budget. In a building expansion, the increases in building gross square feet are supplied by the architect. The hospital must make its own forecast of utilities inflation. Often utilities inflation forecasts can be obtained from the local utility companies, and the analyst can use a national utilities inflation estimate made by one of the major economic institutions or by a government unit.

Housekeeping and maintenance nonsalary expense is adjusted each year for increases in building gross square feet and for inflation. The inflation for these expenses should be forecast at a rate similar to housekeeping and maintenance expense forecasts made by industrial concerns in the hospital's market area. If this cannot be obtained from a board member, the analyst can make an informed estimate by examining forecasted inflation for different components of the government's Consumer Price Index.

Total annual lease expense is normally budgeted separately. An assumption is also needed for total insurance expense that includes costs of malpractice liability insurance; umbrella insurance; fire, theft, and casualty insurance; employee bonding; and any other insurance. These two estimates are often projected in total with no adjustment made for workload changes during the forecast period.

The next assumption in our example is for variable supplies and services per adjusted patient day. This included total nonsalary expenses for all departments not forecast separately. The large items in this category are medical supplies, drugs, pharmaceuticals, food, radiology supplies, disposables, and chemicals. Often one or two of the large items will be culled out and forecast separately. The hospital's historical trend as well as national trends available in the Statistical Abstract of the United States should be used as a guide in forecasting this statistic.

Depreciation expense for major capital improvements should be forecast separately from depreciation for existing and normal replacement assets. Expenditures for major capital construction should be separated into 10-year, 20-year, 30-year, and 40-year components. Depreciation per year for the different component lives are added together to arrive at total depreciation expense by year. It is important to consider all costs before calculating depreciation.

If new construction costs are estimated in current-period dollars, an amount must be added for inflation occurring during the construction term. After total building costs are estimated, several additional costs must be added. These include costs for site development and movable equipment that will depend on the characteristics of the particular construction project. They should also include a reserve and contingency of about ten percent of building costs; professional fees, which may be another ten percent of building costs; and an additional two or three percent of building costs to cover administrative and legal fees.

The next assumption to be made is the amount of capital funds needed for replacement assets. The hospital's fixed asset records are examined to determine the average useful lives of existing assets, and the hospital's historical annual commitment of funds for replacement assets is examined. Using trends determined from these sources, as well as the knowledge gained in the physician interviews, the analyst recommends a forecasted amount by year for replacement assets.

The last assumption is depreciation expense for existing and normal-replacement assets. This is a mathematical exercise that estimates a decreasing annual depreciation on existing assets because of retirements and an increasing annual expense for normal replacement.

Assumptions in Forecasting Working Capital Needs

Working capital is the excess of current assets over current liabilities. The relative amount of working capital gives an indication of the hospital's short-run debt-paying ability. In this section, we will examine ten working capital needs and indicate assumptions and a formula or methodology to forecast each.

The number of days revenue in net receivables is a measure of the collection time lag. With price increases, total dollars in receivables will increase each year. By measuring the number of days revenue in net receivables, the effect of price increases is moderated.

The average number of days of operating expenses in accounts payable is a measure of the processing time to pay nonsalary invoices. The dollar amount of total accounts payable should increase with inflation because the average dollar amount of unpaid invoices will be higher. Shortening the average number of days of operating expenses in accounts payable is normally desirable only if the hospital earns more discounts.

Payroll accruals at year end can be determined as of the end of each year of the forecast by calculating the number of days accrued payroll at each year end and multiplying this by an average day's salary expense. An easier way is to use one half of a pay period and accrue this amount of days for each year of the forecast. This recognizes the very short-lived duration of a payroll accrual amount on a balance sheet.

Annual contributions represent an increase in working capital that does not fluctuate with workloads. Contributions are affected by local and national economic conditions, stability of the local employment market, tax laws, agressiveness of the hospital's development campaign, inflation, and other factors. Predictions based on recent annual historical trends are normally used in long-range forecasting. If the hospital has a definitive plan to solicit funds and the plan will be coordinated by an agency or a person with a past record of successful fund drives, a higher amount may be forecasted. However, assumptions of contribution levels that are significantly higher than the hospital's historical trends are seldom incorporated into feasibility studies because of the uncertainty of the figures.

Interest earnings rate on temporary excess cash should be forecasted conservatively because of the uncertainty associated with this assumption. Other operating revenue is normally forecasted to increase each year at a compound rate equal to inflation. Other operating revenue includes grants, cafeteria income, rental income, income from residency contracts and medical records abstracts, vending machine rebates, television and telephone income, and other miscellaneous revenues.

The last nonpatient revenue assumption to be made is the number of days of reimbursed costs in third party settlements. This will change with increases in the percentage of reimbursed revenue as well as with price increases. If there is a rationale to support a change, the number of days of reimbursed costs is assumed to remain the same throughout the forecast period.

Net Revenue Assumptions

In addition to the expense and the working capital assumptions, the hospital must make several assumptions that directly affect revenue. These are the most complex and at the same time the most critical assumptions to be made. The methodology used and the assumptions made to forecast revenue vary significantly from firm to firm. In this section, we will examine one set of assumptions that can be used effectively to forecast net revenue.

The first patient care assumption that must be made is Medicare and Medicaid revenue as a percentage of total revenue. This percentage is determined by the age and economic status of the population in the service areas as well as by changes in coverage requirements established by these programs. It is anticipated that the percentage of our population that is 65 years of age or older will continue to grow. The scope of services covered by Medicare and Medicaid will continue to grow, and the eligibility requirements to qualify for one of these federal programs will become less restrictive. Because of these factors, Medicare and Medicaid gross revenue as a percentage of total revenue should normally be assumed to increase throughout the forecast period.

The next assumption is percentage of other cost-reimbursed patients to total number of patients. Other cost-reimbursed patients may include those under Blue Cross; county welfare; health maintenance organizations; special arrangements with state, local, or federal agencies; or other entities with which the hospital has cost agreements.

Bad debts, free care, and discounts are normally budgeted as a percentage of gross revenue. Historical and current percentages are examined together to predict these. If there is reason to believe these revenue offsets will decrease because of factors like a more aggressive collection effort, this should be considered in making the forecast. If there is reason to believe these offsets will increase because of things like deteriorating socioeconomic conditions in the hospital's service area, this fact should be incorporated into the forecast.

Average annual price increase per adjusted patient day is predicted tentatively. Revenue generated from hospital price increases is directly related to costs, allowances for contractual adjustments, mix of cost-reimbursed versus charge-reimbursed patients, and other factors. In addition, the hospital must consider the impact of government controls over health care charges to patients. In forecasting price increases, an assumption is put into the simulation model. The net gain or loss is examined, and an adjusted price increase assumption is made. This process is followed until the hospital arrives at a price increase that is reasonable for each year in the forecast period.

The last net revenue assumption to be made involves contractual allowances. It is important that contractual allowances be calculated based on a formula that incorporates the relationship of forecasted gross revenue to forecasted expenses. Some national consulting firms and certified public accounting firms prepare feasibility studies in which contractual allowances are predicted as a stated percentage of gross revenue. This methodology lacks accuracy and may produce a contractual allowance forecast that is significantly inaccurate. In choosing a national firm to prepare a feasibility study, the hospital should examine published official statements to determine how contractual allowances are forecasted by the firm. If they have been estimated as a percentage of gross revenue rather than as a relationship between gross revenue and expenses, the hospital should be aware of the fact that the forecast may contain significant errors.

FINANCIAL PROFORMAS

In previous sections, we examined demand forecasting and the assumption process. These are now used to project financial statements by year.

Planning the Statements

There are two major decisions to make in planning a financial forecast presentation. The first is to decide what years to include. Most forecasts present two years of actual results and five or six years of forecasted statements. Financial forecasting beyond five or six years becomes less reliable because the assumptions made relative to current market conditions, policies of third party payers, the health service environment, and other factors affecting the study are difficult to predict beyond this period. However, if a feasibility study is being performed on a long-range construction project or for a planned expansion that will not begin for several years, forecasts beyond six years should be made. Financial forecasts should extend to two full years of operations after completion of a major expansion or other major change in the hospital's operation. If construction or other change will not be completed for several years, the forecast should be extended to include two full years after completion.

The second major decision to be made in preparing a financial forecast is to choose the statements that will be presented as part of the forecast. All forecasts should include comparative balance sheets, comparative statements of income and expense, and comparative sources and uses of funds. Other statements commonly found in feasibility studies are sources of revenue, sources and uses of construction funds, projected debt service, projected depreciation and amortization, projected cash flow, statements of equity, and other statements applicable to the particular hospital.

Preparing the Statements

A model that takes all of the assumptions made by the analyst and prepares a set of financial statements contains hundreds of calculations. It is not possible to enumerate all of these calculations in this text. We will, however, examine enough of the required calculations to enable the reader to understand some of the complexities inherent in a financial feasibility forecast.

Patient revenue is projected by multiplying the base year by an inflationary factor for increased workload. The product is then multiplied by an inflationary factor for price increases each year. Salaries are forecasted by taking the base year and adjusting it first for an assumed productivity each year, then for number of patient days or other utilization statistic, and finally for an annual increase in the average hourly pay rate. Maintenance, housekeeping, and utilities expenses are adjusted first for projected changes in building gross square feet and then for the assumed inflationary factor for that particular classification of expense. Other expenses are forecasted by year through a series of mathematical calculations. Professional fees per adjusted patient day are predicted by taking the base-period professional fees and adjusting each year for increases in patient days. These amounts are then adjusted for inflation. Variable supplies and services per adjusted patient day are forecasted using this same methodology.

There are four basic principles to remember in forecasting financial statements:

- define a base year
- adjust each year in the forecast for changes in the appropriate workload
- adjust each year in the forecast for inflation
- make sure the mathematical calculations are accumulative and that each year builds upon the previous year—not the base year.

DEBT SERVICE RATIOS

Financial feasibility studies are normally performed to find answers to one of two questions. The first is, Can the hospital service the debt needed to fund a specific, contemplated project? This type of study is normally done in conjunction with an official statement accompanying a bond issue. The second question is, How much debt can the hospital's operations support? This kind of study is normally performed early in a long-range planning effort to enable administration to determine the range of feasible growth. There are many debt service ratios or guidelines that can be used; we will examine here the five ratios that are most frequently used by investment bankers and institutional investors.

Debt to Capitalization

Debt to capitalization is defined as long-term debt divided by long-term debt plus fund balances. As a reasonable comparative measure, this ratio should not exceed 66.6 percent. The formula to express this is:

$$\frac{LTD}{LTD + Eq} \leq 66.6\%$$

where:
LTD is long-term debt
Eq is equity
$\leq$ is less than or equal to

By solving this equation for equity, it can be shown that long-term debt can be as high as three times the amount in the equity section of the balance sheet. This relationship can be used to estimate debt capacity as well as to determine the feasibility of a particular project.

Depreciation Recapture Test

Investment bankers, boards of trustees, and the public are giving increasing importance to this financial test. This is because it is becoming more important for depreciation and amortization recaptured in future years from patient revenues to equal or exceed long-term debt principal payments. This recapture is necessary in the event that federal reimbursement formulas mandate breakeven operating margins that would establish depreciation as the only fund source for principal payments and fixed asset replacements.

Normally depreciation and amortization will significantly exceed loan principal payments in the early years of debt repayment. However, in the later years of debt repayment, when principal payments are greatest, depreciation will normally be significantly less than debt repayment. In calculating projected depreciation and amortization recapture, total depreciation from all hospital assets is compared with total principal requirements from all hospital long-term debt over the life of the loan. This comparative test is illustrated in Table 16–1.

Table 16–1 Community Hospital Depreciation Recapture Test

Estimated Loan Period

Estimated depreciation and amortization from existing assets	$ XX,XXX
Estimated depreciation and amortization from planned new construction	XX,XXX
Total	XXX,XXX
Principal requirements from existing long-term debt	X,XXX
Principal requirements from planned new debt	X,XXX
Total principal requirements	XXX,XXX
Excess (Deficit)	$ XXX

Every time new long-term debt borrowing is contemplated, this calculation should be performed. In a study to project a hospital's new debt capacity or in a study to determine alternative debt repayment periods, appropriate substitutions would be made in the Table 16–1 calculation. The end result should show depreciation and amortization at least equal to loan principal requirements.

Debt to Fixed Assets

The debt-to-fixed-asset calculation assumes that the total long-term borrowing should not exceed 75 percent of fixed asset values. Fixed assets include land, buildings, equipment, and leasehold improvements. Asset cost less depreciation, or book value, is conservatively assumed in many studies to be equal to fixed asset value. Other studies use replacement cost as the value of fixed assets. This practice is not as conservative, but if the other tests are within reasonable limits, replacement cost is acceptable. The formula to determine the debt to fixed asset is:

$$\frac{\text{Projected Long-Term Debt}}{\text{Projected Fixed Asset Value}} \le .75$$

It should be noted that in determining with this test the hospital's ability to support new debt, significant leverage is obtained by not borrowing all of the funds required for a construction project. Every dollar of funds obtained from operations, from fund drives, or from other sources supports additional borrowing.

Debt Service to Operating Expenses

The first of two coverage tests considered important to potential lenders is debt service as a percentage of total operating expenses, where debt service is the total of amortization, depreciation, and interest. A reasonable guideline is that these costs should not exceed ten percent of total expenses. In calculating this ratio, the costs of existing as well as planned new facilities are included. In calculating this coverage ratio, the following can be used as a guide:

Amortization, Depreciation, and Interest Expenses:	
Existing Facilities	$XXX
Planned New Facilities	$XXX
Total	$X,XXX
Total Expenses	$X,XXX

If the hospital's amortization, depreciation, and interest expenses are more than ten percent of total expenses, it is generally regarded as an indication that the hospital has expanded too rapidly.

Debt Service Coverage

Debt service coverage is determined by dividing the first year's principal and interest payments on a long-term loan into the cash that the hospital has available to apply to these payments. Cash available to apply toward debt service is the sum of net income, depreciation and amortization, and interest on long-term debt. An acceptable benchmark is that in the first full year of operation after the new debt, funds available for interest and principal payments should be at least 1–1/2 times debt service. This provides enough funds to make loan payments and also provides a margin for budget errors, normal replacement of existing assets, new technology to meet the needs of increased patient acuity, and other hospital needs.

Analysis of Ratios

The ability of a hospital to incur additional debt is determined by several factors in addition to the five ratio tests we have examined. Some of these factors are local and federal reimbursement policies, the current regulatory environment, the hospital's past profitability, and current market interest rates. The five tests we have reviewed and the generally accepted benchmarks are summarized in Table 16–2.

The Table 16–2 tests should be used only as guides. If the hospital does not meet one or two of the acceptable benchmarks but all other factors are acceptable, financing alternatives may be limited or interest charged may be higher, but the hospital can still obtain borrowed funds. However, if the majority of these benchmarks are not met, the hospital will not be able to borrow funds. It should also be noted that these five financial tests are not all-inclusive. Analysts

Table 16–2 Summary of Ratio Analyses

Financial Tests	Acceptable Benchmarks
Debt to capitalization	Less than 66.6%
Depreciation recapture	At least equal
Debt to fixed assets	Less than 75.0%
Debt service to operating expenses	Less that 10.0%
Debt service coverage	1.5 times

and potential lenders may use many other ratios in addition to or in place of the five shown here.

USE OF THE STUDY

Feasibility studies are normally performed to determine ability to support new debt. The study may be used to determine the kind of debt to be issued, or it may be used as part of the official statement in conjunction with a public offering. In this section we will briefly examine the factors to consider in comparing the different kinds of loans and some considerations of a public offering.

Loan Features

Most hospital long-term debt falls into one of four categories: tax-exempt revenue bonds, taxable bonds, loans insured by the Federal Housing Authority (FHA), and conventional loans.

Tax-exempt revenue bonds are issued through a government agency that has been established to assist hospitals. Most states have passed laws that establish agencies chartered to issue tax-exempt bonds on behalf of tax-exempt hospitals. Proprietary hospitals normally are precluded from borrowing through this agency. The term of a tax-exempt bond issue is negotiable but seldom exceeds 30 years. The terms are negotiable, a performance bond is usually required, and it normally takes 6 months to process the issue and obtain the funds. A feasibility study prepared by an outside firm is required because the only security is a pledge of the hospital's future gross revenues. Although the interest rates on tax-exempt bonds are attractive, there are usually restrictive prepayment penalties during the first 10 years and smaller prepayment penalties after 10 years. Additional bond issues are normally permitted, but it is very expensive to process small bond issues. The hospital normally must borrow more than required for construction in order to fund a debt-service reserve and cover construction interest. This, in effect, increases the effective rate of interest paid on funds used for construction.

Taxable bonds are normally issued for a period of 20 years. The terms of the issue usually require the hospital to meet certain agreed-upon financial covenants. Performance and payment bonding is usually required and the loan-processing time may be from 4 to 5 months. An independent feasibility study may be required, and the loan is secured by a deed of trust in the new property. Prepayment penalties are only one or two percent, and there is normally no prepayment penalty after 5 years. Loan covenants restrict future borrowing options, but refinancing is common if the hospital is prepared to pay substantial refinancing costs.

FHA-insured loans normally have a term of 25 years, and the terms as well as the conditions are dictated. A 100 percent performance and payment bond is required, and the loan application process is complicated. The guidelines and conditions that must be met have made this type of financing unattractive to many hospitals. The loan is secured by a mortgage, but there are normally liberal prepayment privileges available with no penalty. For these loans, the government has extensive design and labor standards, and all construction and architectural documents must have prior approval.

Although a conventional loan normally has a higher interest rate than the other three kinds of loans, it has many attractive advantages. A conventional loan provides maximum flexibility of loan terms with each financing structured to meet the specific needs of the hospital. Of all the alternatives, a conventional loan may be implemented in the shortest time; a three-month processing time is average. An independently prepaid financial feasibility study is normally not required. These loans are normally secured by a deed of trust with a significant prepayment penalty in the first five to ten years. Increases in the loan amount because of cost overruns are relatively easy to obtain.

The above descriptions do not constitute an exhaustive comparison of the four major kinds of borrowing. Our intent here was merely to present the salient points in order to give the reader a basis for comparison. Before entering into any long-term debt of any significance, the hospital administration should seek professional advice to assist in making an informed decision.

The Official Statement

A feasibility study used to support an official statement in a public debt issue is the most comprehensive of all financial feasibility studies. Potential lenders and investment bankers rely on such studies and make decisions based upon them. These investors may be thousands of miles away from the hospital, and the feasibility study is the only means they have of evaluating the merits of the issue. The statements in this type of study are therefore very comprehensive. The study will normally contain from 15 to 25 sections and several appendixes.

In preparing an official statement, the hospital will work with investment bankers, independent public accountants, government agencies, attorneys, and rating agencies such as Moody's or Standard and Poor's. The hospital should choose an investment banking firm in which it has confidence. Because the process is so complicated, the hospital must rely on the skills and judgment of the investment banker or bond underwriter to guide it through the official statement for a public offering.

SUMMARY

Hospital feasibility analyses are performed to determine debt capacity or to prepare for a bond issue or are performed in conjunction with a long-term plan. If the study is part of a public debt issue, the report is most often prepared by a national certified public accounting firm. The hospital should negotiate with the consultants who will work on the study, the amount of work performed by hospital personnel, and other aspects of the engagement. If the study is performed by a consulting firm, the hospital should negotiate the scope of the study and should make a careful analysis of the firm's credentials.

Although there are several advantages to performing a feasibility study with in-house staff, most hospital personnel do not have the experience necessary to complete the study. Moreover, an in-house study may have a lower credibility with the board of directors or potential lenders. Most hospital feasibility studies are performed by a consulting firm or by outside certified public accountants, with some of the work performed by the hospital staff.

Forecasting demand for hospital services is the most critical part of the study. The demand forecast begins with an identification of the hospital's service area. The demographics and social and economic trends of the area are studied. Using projected national or regional norms for hospital usage, the analyst computes a hypothetical demand forecast. This forecast is compared with information obtained in interviews with physicians, area officials, and hospital department heads. Area officials who may be interviewed include major third party payers, hospital administrators, heads of state and local health planning agencies, selected industrial executives, and financial lending executives. Using all of the information gathered, a final estimate of demand for service by year is made.

Before financial statements are prepared, the hospital will need to make many assumptions that affect the statements. The expense assumptions are used to forecast the hospital's operating expenses by year at the estimated level of activity predicted in the demand analysis. It is necessary to forecast working capital needs to ensure an adequate cash flow and to give an indication of the hospital's short-run, debt-paying ability. In addition to the expense and working capital assumptions, the hospital must make several assumptions that directly affect revenue. These are the most complex and at the same time the most critical of the assumptions that must be made.

Although there are many ratios and guidelines that can be used to determine the hospital's ability to support additional debt, there are five that are most frequently used by potential lenders. The ratios or guidelines are debt to capitalization, depreciation recapture, debt to fixed assets, debt service to operating expenses, and debt service coverage. These tests should be used only as guides. Other factors as well as other tests are also important.

Most hospital long-term debt falls into one of four categories: Tax-exempt revenue bonds have an attractive interest rate, but there are several disadvantages to this type of borrowing. Taxable bonds normally have several restrictive covenants. FHA-insured loans involve a complicated application process, and there are many guidelines and conditions that must be met. A conventional loan normally has a high interest rate. Each of these four kinds of borrowing has advantages and disadvantages. Professional advice should be obtained before entering into any significant long-term debt agreement.

DISCUSSION QUESTIONS

1. Name some of the items that a national certified public accounting firm may require before accepting a contract to do a financial feasibility study for a hospital. Explain the rationale for these requirements.
2. What are some of the advantages of having extensive hospital staff involvement in the preparation of a financial feasibility study?
3. Who are some area officials who may be interviewed in a financial feasibility study? How do such interviews contribute to the accuracy of the study?
4. List some assumptions that must be made in a financial feasibility analysis.
5. How should contractual allowances be calculated in a forecast?
6. Explain the two major decisions that must be made in planning a financial forecast presentation.
7. What are the four basic principles to remember in forecasting financial statements?
8. Define the five ratios most commonly used to determine a hospital's debt capacity.
9. Compare tax-exempt revenue bonds with taxable bonds issued by the hospital.
10. What is an official statement? How is it used?

Index

283

Self-pay receivables, 65–70
  collection of, 68
Seminars for new employees, 84
Sensitivity analysis, 221
Separation of duties, 40–41
Service area, 262–263
Service bureaus, 205
Service goals, 5
Shared computer services, 204
Shifting of costs, 66–67, 145
SHUR. *See* System of Hospital Uniform Reporting
Sick leave, 36–37
Signature plates, 25, 41, 164
Silver recovery revenue, 59, 111, 142
Simulation, 221
  defined, 215
Social goals, 5
Social responsibilities, 5
Social Security, 32, 37, 238
Social service department, 67
Software, defined, 215
Source document, defined, 215
Sources of cash, 120, 122, 237, 240–241, 242, 245–248
Specific identification method of inventory pricing, 185
Speculative motive for holding cash, 243
Staffing, 53, 55, 225
  See also Employees; Payroll; Personnel
Standardization of hospital accounting, 3
State governments, 3
State and local government securities, 244
State and local taxes, 33, 38
Statement of income, 122, 140
Statistical assumptions, 80
Statistical budgets, 97, 119, 125–126, 126
Statistical forecast worksheet, 100
Statistical information standardization, 3
Statistics
  comparative patient-day, 98
  distribution, 117

historical patient-day, 97
operating, 125
reporting of, 123
unit cost, 122
workload, 125
Statutes of limitation, 31
Step-down process, 103, 104, 143
Stocking, 175–177
  See also Inventory
Stockout, 176
Storage in computers, 197–198
Subobjectives, 218
Subsystem, defined, 215
Supervisor of accounting, 1
Supplies
  budgeting for, 239–240
  expense for, 125
  service area for, 263
  wasted, 47
Supporting schedules, 124–125
Surgery and computers, 190
Suspense accounts, 57
System of Hospital Uniform Reporting (SHUR), 2, 3

T

Taxable bonds, 279
Taxes, 251–256
  state and local, 33, 38
  unemployment, 32–33
  withholding. *See* Withholding taxes
Tax-exempt organizations, 251–253
Tax reports, 29
Tax-sheltered annuity program, 36
Technology, 6, 101, 139
Telephone collections, 68
Telephone revenue, 111, 119, 142, 272
Television rental revenue, 111, 142, 272
Temporary employees, 42
Temporary investments, 42, 243–245
Temporary sources of cash, 245–248
Terminals, defined, 215
Termination clause in contract, 228
Termination of employees, 41

About the Author

DONALD F. BECK, M.B.A., C.P.A., is the controller of one of the largest not-for-profit hospital systems in the United States. He has worked in small hospitals for a large proprietary chain and as financial officer for a noted regional medical center in the Midwest. Mr. Beck has taught college accounting and finance and is a frequent lecturer before professional groups. He has chaired seminars for the American Institute of Certified Public Accountants, American Management Associations, hospitals and hospital associations, colleges, universities, and other organizations. He is the author of several articles and has served as financial consultant to numerous hospitals on reimbursement, budgeting, cost accounting, data processing applications, and financial forecasting.